QUALITY IN PATIENT CARE INC

Abstract

Straightforward simple and easy-to-understand information tailored for daily patient care with a special section dedicated to the care of geriatric patients focused on managing patients with dementia.

Gladys N Jusino Leon, DNP, MSN, RN, CMSRN, GERO-BC

INTRODUCTION

My nursing career, which has spanned over thirty years, has been driven by a deep passion. I have always been committed to alleviating pain and delivering the compassionate care I wish for my family and friends. I've served in diverse settings and specialized units, continually enriching my expertise and understanding. However, the most profound influence on my life in recent years was witnessing my father endure inadequate care at the hands of unqualified and careless healthcare providers.

In November 2022, my father endured a hemorrhagic stroke and was moved to a larger hospital, which had limited staff and resources. Within five days, he developed a urinary tract infection, pneumonia, influenza, multiple pressure sores, and a fungal infection in his mouth and other areas. The neurology team opted to discontinue his care without informing me. He was not given any nourishment, and no one addressed the secretions accumulating until I intervened, requesting oxygen and suction, which I administered myself due to the absence of nursing care, aside from initiating the necessary IV antibiotics. There was no communication regarding his care plan, test results, or the medications being given.

Services did not include perineal care, catheter care, oral care, bed baths, or repositioning during that period. Responses to inquiries were limited to "The oxygen concentrator is broken, but I know how much oxygen he is receiving by the bubbles in the humidifier" or there was an evident absence of knowledge, accountability, concern, and compassion.

After spending 14 days on a stretcher in the emergency department and developing numerous wounds, I finally managed to transfer my father to a nursing home. However, he required a feeding tube. Before its placement, he endured another 14 days in a different hospital due to sepsis from inadequate care. Following the feeding tube insertion and on the day of his discharge, a nurse improperly administered medication, leading to my father's pulmonary aspiration. This nurse failed to introduce himself to my father or me, acknowledge us, heed my warnings about repositioning, or make eye contact. He washed his hands and exited the room. Five days later, my father passed away. He was 94 years old.

The difficulties encountered in the healthcare system led to the creation of Quality in Patient Care Inc., a non-profit organization legally recognized in Georgia and Puerto Rico and federally certified as a 501(c)3 entity. Its mission is to strengthen healthcare facilities and clinical staff, ensure the delivery of quality healthcare services by promoting professional growth through education and training, and build the essential infrastructure to support these endeavors.

I have become clear that I need to write a book. Many medical and surgical textbooks for nurses contain intricate and complex material. Presenting this information straightforwardly and factually will improve educational results, making it easier for nursing and allied health students and professionals to learn and retain knowledge for the long term.

I desire that this book becomes a valuable resource for expanding your knowledge and comprehension of medical and surgical nursing.

PRESENTATION OF THE INFORMATION

Understanding the fundamental aspects of body systems is crucial for general and specialized care in acute and chronic conditions. This knowledge enables nurses to foster healthier outcomes for patients with impaired bodily functions, recognize the signs and symptoms that warrant reporting to a primary care provider, and implement appropriate interventions for chronic conditions within their nursing practice scope.

Each chapter will initially detail a body system's basic structure and function. It will also describe age-related changes and prevalent chronic conditions associated with that system. Moreover, diagnostic tests and procedures easily supplement general information on the body system. Diagnostic tests and procedures play a crucial role in detecting and identifying diseases. These tests are essential for monitoring—the progression-and evaluation of the effectiveness of the treatments to manage or cure the disease. Clinical manifestations and anticipated treatments will follow. Finalizing the chapter with nursing interventions to achieve the best possible patient outcomes.

OCCASIONALLY A TEXT BOX WILL APPEAR TO EMPHASIZE IMPORTANT INFORMATION FOUND IN THE CHAPTER.

Chapter eleven presents information on gerontological nursing, aging changes, and precise interventions related to those normal changes and other prevalent changes expected to occur in older adults.

NURSING PRACTICE AND PROFESSIONALISM

4

NURSING PRACTICE AND PROFESSIONALISM

The word nurse is a variant of the Latin word *nutricius*, which means nourish. However, the word nurse refers to service. A nurse is a healthcare professional trained to care for and assist an individual who is physically sick or who has succumbed to illness. Nurses care for people who are vulnerable, fragile, and unable to care for themselves. A nurse is someone who demonstrates competency when providing care.

The nursing code of ethics guides "carrying out nursing responsibilities in a manner consistent with quality in nursing care and the ethical obligations of the profession." Ethics are a set of moral values or principles that guide behavior. Ethical behavior and professionalism in nursing go together. Ethics is the philosophy and discipline dealing with what is good and bad. It is often referred to in context with moral duty and obligation.

Professionalism is the quality that characterizes a professional person. A person is referred to as being "professional" when the ethical standards of a profession characterize the person's behavior. Professionalism is not something that is "worn" occasionally. Professionalism is an integral part of the person, with the person behaving in a professional way all the time.

> "ETHICAL BEHAVIOR IS DOING THE RIGHT THING WHEN NO ONE ELSE IS WATCHING—EVEN WHEN DOING THE WRONG THING IS LEGAL."
>
> McMillan, 2018

Ethics and professionalism are important traits to maintain integrity and credibility in the workplace. In 2020, 89% of adults in the United States rated nursing as the #1 most trusted profession. Nursing has been chosen as the #1 most trusted profession for the 22nd year in a row for a reason. However, only 78% of adults in the United States now believe nurses have "very high" or "high" honesty and ethical standards. Why this decline?

This decline may be related to nurses lowering their standards and providing a lesser quality of care, with patients and families not being at the center of the care. There are many reasons for this change in behavior and attitude at the bedside. Regardless of the reasons, nurses commit to humanity the moment they complete their education and training.

Character

The word "character" defines a person with unique qualities that distinguish or set him or her apart from everybody else. A person described as "a person of character" presents good qualities, including moral and ethical principles, emotional strength, honesty, and fairness. Having a "good character" is a phrase used to indicate that the individual is someone whose opinion is considered essential and a person of his or her word.

Communication and Nursing Practice

Communication impacts nurse-patient relations, influencing patient satisfaction. It also impacts nurse-to-nurse communication, elevating coworkers' relations and enhancing teamwork. Effective communication promotes high-quality nursing care and patient safety. Communication impacts nurse-patient relations, influencing patient satisfaction. Nurses who communicate well will understand the patient's culture, helping them provide patient-centered care. Communication also influences clinical reasoning and decision-making, promoting effective health care and positive patient outcomes. Communication with the healthcare team is necessary to provide effective patient care. Effective communication helps the nurse perform detailed patient assessment, identifying critical physical and psychosocial issues affecting the patient holistically. Good communication skills in nursing practice prevent errors in patient care through verbal communication, body language, and documentation. Healthcare professionals with good communication skills can become better patient advocates.

Emotional Competence and Professionalism

"Emotional competence is the demonstration of self-efficacy in emotion-eliciting social transactions" (Bar-On & Parker, 2000, p. 68). Self-efficacy translates cultural values and beliefs into self-personal thoughts and behavior. These qualities are demonstrated in how the individual expresses his or her emotions in interactions with others (socially) to advance toward desired outcomes or goals. Mature emotional competence promotes personal integrity by integrating moral character, ethical principles, and values, influencing emotional responses. Today's healthcare system is characterized by constant change and competitive pressures, and emotional competence and social qualities are essential. Leadership in the healthcare system today is also motivated to improve employees' expertise to promote organizational productivity and competitiveness. Social and emotional qualities necessary to be successful include self-confidence, flexibility, persistence, empathy, and the ability to get along with others. These attributes are linked to superior performance. Other social and emotional competencies employers look for in nurses are personal self and time management, motivation to set goals, adaptability to increased practice changes, teamwork and interpersonal effectiveness, and leadership potential qualities.

Summary

Professional behavior is demonstrated through how the person speaks, behaves, looks, and leads, including attitudes, body language, and nonverbal communication. Principles of professionalism include:

- Being polite and treating others with respect
- Being ethical and honest
- Making sound decisions
- Presenting a positive attitude

- Dressing appropriately
- Following the corporation's policies and procedures
- Arriving at work a few minutes early
- Taking responsibility for your actions
- Being reliable and responsible
- Good communication skills
- Asking for help during difficult situations
- Being trustworthy
- Helping others
- Looking for ways to improve
- Avoid gossip and foul language
- Be careful with social media and posts related to work
- Be cautious about oversharing

CHAPTER 1

THE CARDIAC SYSTEM

The cardiovascular system is vital for transporting oxygen and nutrients throughout the body and for removing waste. This system consists of the heart, arteries, veins, and capillaries, which are fundamental to cellular function. Managing blood pressure and cholesterol levels is essential to maintaining the body's homeostasis and metabolism in optimal condition. Heart health is crucial and can be maintained through regular exercise, and a balanced diet.

DIAGNOSTIC LABS

Erythromycin Sedimentation Rate (ESR) – This blood test identifies if there is any inflammation process in the body. Inflammation is the immune system's response to injury, infection, or abnormal conditions that appear in the body. However, it does not specify the location. The result of this test increases when the myocardial muscle is damaged.

Blood Urea Nitrogen (BUN) and creatinine (Cr)—The BUN measures the amount of urea nitrogen in the blood. Urea nitrogen and creatinine are waste products eliminated through the kidneys. Finding them in the blood indicates that the kidneys are not functioning well. An increased level of these waste products is related to the poor prognosis of patients with CHF. If the heart is not functioning adequately, kidney function will become impaired.

CPK-MB – Creatine Phosphokinase-MB is an enzyme released by the heart (cardiac enzyme) when the heart muscle is damaged (such as when a person suffers a heart attack), becoming elevated in the blood, this test is ordered to identify heart muscle damage (MB) versus skeletal muscle damage (MM).

Troponin I – Troponin is a myocardial protein that becomes elevated when the heart muscle is damaged.- It elevates at about the same time as the CPK-MB enzyme and stays in the blood for weeks.

HIGH TRIGLYCERIDES + HIGH LDL = HEART ATTACK

LDH (Lactate Dehydrogenase), SGOT (Glutamic-Oxaloacetic Transaminase), AST (Aspartate Aminotransferase), ALT (Alanine Aminotransferase), and ALP (Alkaline Phosphatase) – These enzymes leak into the bloodstream when the liver is inflamed or damaged. High levels of ALT, AST, and ALP in blood could indicate conditions like fatty liver, hepatitis, or cirrhosis. ALT is found in liver cells. High levels in the blood indicate damage to liver cells. AST is found in liver and heart muscle cells. A high level could indicate heart cell damage. ALP is found in bones and the liver. High levels of ALP may indicate liver, bone, or gallbladder problems. LDH becomes elevated several hours after cardiac muscle damage.

Cholesterol – Cholesterol is a fatty-like substance found in cells and is used to complete some cellular processes. The cholesterol levels should be <200mg/dL for adults and <170mg/dL for children.

> LDL (*Low-Density Lipoprotein* = "bad cholesterol") – The average level should be <100mg/dL. High levels put the person at risk for heart disease and stroke.
>
> HDL – (*High-Density Lipoprotein* = "good cholesterol) This is the cholesterol that removes the "bad cholesterol" (LDL) from the bloodstream, carrying it to the liver to be discarded from the body. The average level should be <40mg/dL.

Triglycerides – Not-used calories are converted into triglycerides (fat). The fat is then stored in the fat cells and used later and between meals. The average level should be <150mg/dL.

C-reactive protein (CRP)—The liver makes this when an injury or infection occurs, causing inflammation inside the body. Inflammation is associated with atherosclerosis, or the buildup of plaques in the arteries. This test helps identify the risk of heart disease.

DIAGNOSTIC TESTS

Swan-Ganz – Another name for this catheter is pulmonary artery catheter. The Swan-Ganz is a catheter that helps get the information needed to diagnose a heart or lung issue and determine treatment. It is used to identify how well the blood moves and is especially important to identify right and left CHF. No complications are expected, but medications can help relax the patient while the catheter is placed. This test helps indicate the filling pressure in the left and right ventricles, the pressure in the pulmonary artery, and cardiac output. Remember to deflate the balloon after each reading.

Cardiac Catheterization (Angiogram) – This is the insertion of a catheter into an artery, usually the femoral artery, to instill a dye to view coronary vessels. It is used to identify occluded/blocked coronary vessels. Before the procedure, distal pulses and dye allergy, VS, and voids must be assessed and marked. Patients may be asked to cough to clear dye from arteries and disrupt any dysrhythmias during the procedure. After the procedure, assess the distal pulse, check the site, and VS. Keep the patient flat or in a low Fowler's position if there is a respiratory problem, with the affected extremity in extension for six hours. Patients will be instructed to continue light activity for two weeks.

PTCA (Percutaneous Transluminal Coronary Angioplasty) – The PTCA involves inserting a balloon catheter into an artery to dilate the occluded coronary vessel. It is an alternative to Open Heart Surgery and follows the same process indicated if administered during the procedure or cardiac catheterization. The sheath is removed from heparin during the procedure when the PTT level is acceptable. It is important to assess the distal pulse after the procedure.

EKG (*Electrocardiogram)*: This noninvasive test is used to identify arrhythmias, the effectiveness of medications, and MI (it will show an elevated ST segment). It is a priority when multiple premature ventricular contractions (PVCs) are identified. Although these irregular heartbeats are common and not usually dangerous, the patient is at risk for complications when there are other comorbidities, such as congenital heart disease. If PVCs continue, the heart muscle will weaken, causing cardiomyopathy.

Stress Test—Also known as Exercise EKG. The patient remains NPO for four hours. While connected to an EKG, the patient is monitored while walking on a treadmill. Reassure the patient that the test will be stopped if chest pain develops.

The Thallium Stress Test - This imaging test, also called a nuclear stress test is done when a patient cannot walk. Instead of exercising on the treadmill, patients receive vasodilators such as Persantine and a radioactive tracer called Thallium. EKG is monitored as thallium is given using ultrasound to show images of the heart. The purpose of this test is to see if perfusion of thallium occurs after vasodilation. If thallium is not observed, there is an occlusion.

TEE (Transesophageal Echocardiogram) – This invasive test detects and evaluates the severity of coronary artery disease by using sound waves to create pictures of the heart. It identifies blocked (clots) in coronary vessels, aneurysms, cancer tumors, and endocarditis. Before the test, the patient stays NPO for six hours and receives IV sedation and anesthesia. After the test the remain NPO for four hours. Patients will receive warm liquids when the gag reflex returns.

CONDITIONS

MYOCARDIAL INFARCTION (MI; Heart Attack)

This condition is caused by impaired blood flow caused by thrombus, embolus, spasm, and cocaine. Signs and symptoms are chest pain (*angina*), cool diaphoresis (sweating), low BP, pallor (ashen color), restlessness, nausea, and vomiting. It is diagnosed by an elevated ST segment on the EKG and increased CPK-MB and Troponin levels.

The patient is placed in a semi-Fowler's position to decrease the heart's preload (workload). To begin anticoagulation, the patient receives aspirin. The preferred vasodilator is *Nitroglycerin*, but sometimes patients receive Morphine Sulfate IVP (IV push) to dilate coronary vessels and reduce pain by decreasing myocardial oxygen demand.

Lidocaine is the antiarrhythmic medication used. Heparin is administered if a patient has had pain for over six hours. If the pain has developed in less than six hours, the physician will prescribe *Agrastat* with heparin or tPA. Oxygen is delivered at 2L via nasal cannula.

Agrastat - anticoagulation medication given to patients with severe chest pain or patients undergoing angioplasty. This medication is also used to treat early neurological deterioration after a stroke.

ACE Inhibitors—These medications decrease myocardial oxygen demand by increasing water and sodium excretion from the kidneys. When these medications are given, monitor K levels (potassium). Do not give these medications to renal patients.

HOW TO PERFORM THE VALSALVA MANEUVER

1. SIT DOWN OR LIE ON YOUR BACK.
2. TAKE A BREATH.
3. PUSH THAT BREATH OUT AGAINST YOUR CLOSED MOUTH AND NOSE WHILE STRAINING AS IF YOU'RE TRYING TO HAVE A BOWEL MOVEMENT.
4. HOLD FOR 15 TO 20 SECONDS.

Lidocaine—this medication is used to treat arrhythmias related to potassium imbalances. When this medication is given, assess for signs and symptoms of neurotoxicity, such as confusion, headache, tremors, or blurred vision.

Patients should follow a low-cholesterol and low-sodium diet. They should avoid processed foods like cold cuts, hot dogs, instant pudding, canned soups, ham, pork, smoked meats, avocado, and celery. Patients will also be placed in cardiac rehabilitation. Pain relief is a priority for these patients.

Avoid performing the *Valsalva Maneuver*. The Valsalva Maneuver is a breathing technique used to diagnose problems associated with the autonomic nervous system. Patients with arrhythmias like supraventricular tachycardia (SVT) use this technique to restore a standard heart rate. Patients should avoid using this technique after an MI.

ANGINA PECTORIS (Chest Pain)

When the circulation (blood flow) to the heart muscle is compromised, the patient will experience chest pain called angina. Blood flow to the heart muscle can be compromised by 4 E's: Exercise, Eating, Excitement (stress/emotions), or Environment (cold). Smoking is also a factor that puts people at risk for angina and cardiac events. Signs and symptoms are chest pain that subsides with rest. The physician will administer medications if an EKG reveals more than six PVC in one minute. Some medicines that are frequently given to patients experiencing angina are aspirin and nitroglycerin (NTG). Nitroglycerin tablets are sublingual (SL). The patient can receive one tablet every five minutes and up to three tablets. The patient will experience tingling under the tongue when this medication is given.

Another way to administer NTG is through a *Nitro-Dur Transdermal* patch. Nitro patches should be applied with gloves to avoid absorbing the medication. Place the hand on the hairless chest or upper arm for ten seconds to enhance absorption. Wash off old sites with soap and water before applying a new patch to a new site. If the patient develops angina while on the Nitro patch, give nitroglycerin tablets as indicated above.

Patients' education includes sex precautions for cardiac patients. The patient should be in a dependent position. An NTG tablet should be taken before sexual activity. It is acceptable for the patient to have sex when they can take one flight of stairs without experiencing shortness of breath (SOB). Cardiac patients should walk at a slow pace and rest. Diet is the same as for MI patients.

CONGESTIVE HEART FAILURE (CHF)

Congestive heart failure develops in patients who have experienced MI, atherosclerosis heart disease (ASHD), myopathy, thyroid storm, fever, anemia, and acidosis.

	Right CHF	Left CHF
Description	Venous side-R atrium-CHF congestion	Arterial side – Lung congestion PRIORITY
Manifestation	Jugular Vein Distension (JVD)=Neck vein congestion Hepatomegaly (Enlarged liver)	Pulmonary edema=Crackles (rales) lung sounds

Signs and Symptoms	Cold edema in legs Abdominal distension	Dyspnea, SOB, orthopnea, cyanosis Cough with pink, frothy sputum
Assessment	Number of pillows the patient sleeps with at night=Orthopnea	
Treatment	3 D's: Digoxin, Dilators, Diuretics. Digoxin is also a diuretic. For R-CHF, keep your legs up higher than your waist level. For L-CHF, keep your legs in an extension or a dependent position.	
Nursing	Check I&O, daily weight, and fluid restriction. Monitor potassium and sodium levels. Maintain the patient in a semi-fowler's position. Administer oxygen 2-3L/NC. Assess for fluid/volume excess, activity intolerance, and impaired gas exchange.	

Digoxin level = 0.5-2.0 ng/dL. Assess for signs of toxicity. These include anorexia, nausea, vomiting, vision impairment, bradycardia, and diarrhea. The antidote used is Digibind. Remember the 3 Ds related to digoxin toxicity: Digoxin, Diarrhea, and *Digibind.*

The diuretic used is Spironolactone (Aldactone). Lasix is not used because it will decrease the potassium level in the system. If used, it is important to monitor the potassium level often.

CARDIAC TAMPONADE

This condition is related to pericardial effusion, which compresses the heart due to fluid build-up in the pericardium. A vital intervention related to this condition is to assess for shortness of breath, cough, muffled heart sounds, and pulse paradoxes. Pulsus paradoxus occurs when the BP and pulse rate fall during inspiration. The common causes are pericardial effusion, pleural effusion, or when the pericardium becomes stiff, asthma, COPD, or pneumothorax.

> PULSUS PARADOXUS IS A SUDDEN DROP IN BLOOD PRESSURE, SPECIFICALLY SYSTOLIC BLOOD PRESSURE, WHEN THE PATIENT IS BREATHING (INHALING), WHICH AFFECTS THE AMOUNT OF OXYGEN THE CELLS RECEIVE.
>
> Hamzaoui, Monnet, and Teboul, 2013

PACEMAKER

A pacemaker regulates the heart rate. It is a battery-powered device placed under the skin near the collarbone to prevent bradycardia or a slow heartbeat. There are three types: single-chamber, dual-chamber, and biventricular. The single-chamber pacemaker sends signals to the heart's lower right chamber (right ventricle). The dual-chamber pacemaker sends signals to the heart's upper and lower right chambers (right atrium and ventricle). The biventricular pacemaker, also called a resynchronization pacemaker, stimulates the two lower chambers (right and left ventricles), strengthening the heart muscle. Pacemakers can also be temporary or permanent.

Temporary

These are *external pacemakers*. The patient's arm closest to the site has decreased movement. If the patient needs to be defibrillated, do not defibrillate over the lead wire site. Securely tape the wires to the chest.

Permanent

Permanent pacemakers are *internal.* The patient will have decreased activity of the arm closest to the site for 48 to 72 hours. Education includes electrical safety instructions. Patients should avoid using cellphones, microwaves, electric garage door openers, short wave radios, MRI, and store/airport security devices (do not scan directly over the site). No contact sports. It is a good idea to wear a medic-alert identification tag.

Automatic Implantable Cardioverter Defibrillator (AICD)

This device detects and ends life-threatening events such as *ventricular tachycardia, ventricular fibrillation, and sudden death syndrome*. Nursing care involves everything discussed in the pacemaker section. Educate patients to avoid heavy lifting.

Cardiopulmonary Resuscitation (CPR)

Assess the patient by looking and listening for breathing. Feel for the pulse. No pulse? Call a code, do not leave the patient, and start CPR. For an adult, the compressions-to-breathes ratio is 30-2. The goal is to complete 80-120 compressions/minute. Compressions should be 2" deep.

PERIPHERAL VASCULAR DISEASE (PVD)

Intermittent claudication is the main symptom of PVD. When *Intermittent Claudication* occurs, the patient experiences pain in the lower extremities while walking. Gravity pulls down blood vessels to the feet. When the pain occurs, the patient should be instructed to stop, remain standing, or rest and continue walking. Progressive walking will prevent the worsening of impaired circulation.

Arterial Disease – A type of PVD affecting specifically the arteries of either extremities, upper or lower. It differs from venous disease because the pain experienced in the lower extremities will go away when the person is at rest and keeping <u>legs extended</u> but not elevated. If the person develops ulcers, they are more common on the legs and feet. Signs and symptoms of the arterial condition include erectile dysfunction, wasting of leg muscles, and leg discoloration.

Venous Disease – In this type of PVD, when the patient experiences pain, the lower extremities must be elevated. In addition, varicose veins and ulcers developed on the ankles distinguish arterial PVD from venous disease. The signs and symptoms of the condition affecting the veins include leg swelling, pain, heaviness, and skin darkening.

HYPERTENSION (HTN)

Hypertension is diagnosed when a patient's BP is consistently >120/80 or at least on two separate occasions. Primary hypertension is when there is no known cause. Retake the BP 15 minutes later if the patient has no other symptoms. Manual BP is recommended.

Risk factors are smokers, obesity, stress, diabetes, heart disease, and people in sitting jobs. African Americans are at risk for developing hypertension. Diet plays a significant role in controlling and modifying HTN. Patients should follow a low-cholesterol and low-sodium diet. Teach the patient to rise slowly to prevent experiencing what is called *postural hypertension.* Exercise is important. Also, losing weight is essential to control HTN and help decrease any dyspnea (difficulty breathing) the patient may present.

Medications include beta-blockers (ending on "olol"), ACE inhibitors (ending on "pril"), diuretics (Lasix, Bumex, Esidrix), Aldactone (potassium-sparing diuretic), and thiazides (lose potassium). It is essential to monitor potassium levels whenever the patient is on diuretics and monitor weight daily.

EFFECTIVE CARDIOVERSION

Cardioversion is used for severe atrial fibrillation that does not respond to medications (digoxin, calcium channel blockers, quinidine, and procainamide). Before performing cardioversion, the patient needs to remain on NPO for six hours and hold digoxin for 48 hours. After the procedure, monitoring the airway is a priority. Check vital signs and oxygen saturation levels and monitor EKG.

PULSE ASSESSMENT AND ARRHYTHMIAS

Pulse Assessment/Pulse Deficit

1. Assess the apical pulse.
2. If the patient presents irregular pulse, assess for pulse deficit. - Take radial and apical pulses simultaneously and note rate and rhythm. Pulse deficit is expected in atrial flutter and atrial fibrillation.

Atrial Fibrillation (Most common dysrhythmia)

Atrial Fibrillation (AFib) is a rapid atrial and ventricular rate-like atrial flutter. The EKG will show irregular indiscernible P waves referred to as F waves (fibrillatory waves). Risk factors include hypertension, cardiomyopathy, hyperthyroidism, pulmonary disease, and alcohol. Some signs and symptoms to expect are pulse deficit, palpitations, fatigue, and malaise.

Atrial fibrillation usually converts to *normal sinus rhythm* (NSR) without treatment within 24 hours. If not, cardioversion should be used within 48 hours. To prevent embolus formation, the medications used to convert atrial fibrillation back to NSR are IV Adenosine, PO Quinidine, Amiodarone, or Procainamide, and blood thinners.

ATRIAL FIBRILLATION HAS A HIGH RISK FOR EMBOLUS FORMATION CAUSING CVA. EXPECT THE PATIENT TO RECEIVE BLOOD THINNER MEDICATION. THIS MEDICATION CANNOT BE STOPPED WITHOUT MEDICAL ADVICE.

Atrial flutter causes a therapeutic block at the AV node. The EKG will present a sawtooth P wave called a *fibrillatory wave* (F wave). Classical signs and symptoms include chest pain, the first symptom, shortness of breath, hypotension, and pulse deficit. Like AFib, the treatment of atrial flutter is cardioversion or medications to convert to NSR. The same medicines mentioned for atrial fibrillation are used. If stable and there is no cardioversion, the patient will receive calcium blockers (Diltiazem) or verapamil (Calan), Beta Blockers ("olol"), and Digoxin. These medications are given to decrease the ventricular rate and AV node rate.

An abdominal aneurysm extends through the abdomen. When an area on the aorta's wall becomes weak and unable to manage the pressure of blood pumping from the heart, the weak area enlarges. Factors like aging, tobacco use, and certain medical conditions can weaken the aorta's wall. Other risk factors include being Caucasian, 60 to 90 years old, history of HTN, and atherosclerosis. The signs and symptoms include pulsatile abdominal mass, systolic bruit over mass, and severe back or abdominal pain signifying rupture. The patient will require surgery when the weak area of the abdominal aorta is >2 inches (5cm) in diameter.

Coronary Artery Disease (CAD) – A person develops CAD when fat and fibrous tissue develops inside the cardiac arteries (atherosclerosis), blocking and narrowing the vessels and decreasing blood flow to the heart. Risk factors include African American descent, age, male gender (three times more likely than females), and family history. There are modifiable risk factors such as hypertension, diabetes, smoking, obesity, high LDL, low HDL, lack of exercise, and lack of estrogen in women.

Femoral Popliteal Bypass – The femoral artery is the largest in the thigh, providing blood to the leg. When the artery becomes diseased and sclerosed, this procedure is performed to reroute blood flow in the legs due to arterial insufficiency, causing intermittent claudication). The same risk factors included under the coronary artery disease (CAD) section apply to this condition.

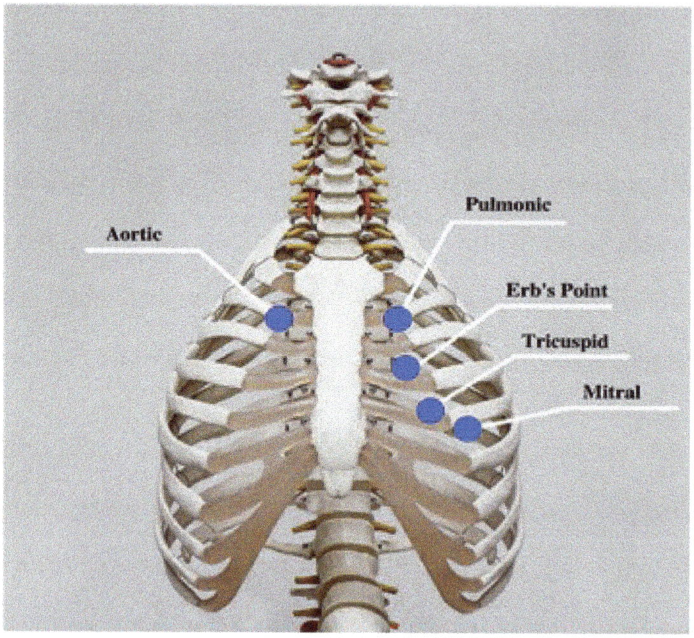

CARDIAC LANDMARKS	
Aorta	Second intercostal space right of sternum
Pulmonic Area	Second intercostal space to left of sternum
Erb's Point	Third intercostal space to left of sternum
Tricuspid Area	Right Ventricle – Fourth intercostal space to the left of the sternum
Apical Area	Left Ventricle – Fifth intercostal space to left of the sternum, Midclavicular
Point of Maximal Impulse (PMI)	Location of the chest wall where heart contractions can be palpated, usually on the left of the sternum fifth intercostal space at the midclavicular line. It may be found right below the nipple.

CARDIAC MEDICATIONS

CARDIAC MEDICATIONS					
MEDICATION	EXAMPLES	ACTION	USE	ADVERSE REACTION	RECOMMENDATIONS
Beta Blockers (Antagonists)	"ol, olol, alol" Propanolol Labetalol	Decrease heart rate, BP, and contractility.	Hypertension Angina MI	Fatigue, orthostatic hypotension, dizziness, bradycardia, CHF,	Please do not use it with oral hypoglycemics or bronchodilators.

	Metoprolol Pindolol Nadolol Atenolol Carvedilol		Sometimes CHF	and hypoglycemia (which mask symptoms) may increase airway resistance.	Do not give to asthmatic patients. Give with food. Nephrotoxic. Avoid hot baths or saunas related to hypotensive risk.
Alpha Blockers (Antagonists)	"zosin" Doxazosin Prazosin Terazosin	Acts on peripheral vasculature to reduce peripheral vascular resistance and produce vasodilation	Hypertension BPH (Benign Prostate Hyperplasia)	Orthostatic hypotension, edema, tachycardia, rhinitis, vision changes, decreased WBC.	Do not use in patients with liver disease.
Calcium Channel Blockers (Antagonists)	"dipines" Amlodipine Nifedipine Nimodipine Felodipine Nicardipine Diltiazem Verapamil	Inhibits calcium ion influx across cardiac smooth muscle cells, decreasing contractility and oxygen demand. Decreases apical pulse and BP.	Hypertension Angina	Dizziness, weakness, peripheral edema, hypotension, MI, heart failure, nasal congestion, cough, pulmonary edema, muscle cramps, constipation	Do not use Beta Blockers with this medication because it will put the patient at risk for hypotension and CHF. Do not use Ginko or Ginseng because it will bring increased CBC effects and toxicity. Do not give sublingual because it will cause severe hypotension, MI, and death.
ACE Inhibitors	"pril, ril, vil" Captopril Ramipril Enalapril Accupril Quinapril Lisinopril Benazepril	It prevents angiotensin I from converting to angiotensin II, blocking vasoconstriction. Less angiotensin II decreases peripheral arterial resistance, decreases aldosterone secretion, reduces sodium and water retention, and lowers BP.	Hypertension CHF Post MI	Hypotension, tachycardia, dizziness, fainting, decreased CBC values, hyperkalemia.	These medications should not be given with NSAIDs because NSAIDs will block the effect of ACE, potassium-sparing, and diuretics/supplements. Separate administration of antacids by one to two hours. Do not give to renal failure patients. Take on an empty stomach (1 hr. before meals).

CARDIAC MEDICATIONS					
MEDICATION	EXAMPLES	ACTION	USE	ADVERSE REACTION	RECOMMENDATIONS
ACE II Inhibitors (Angiotensin Receptor Blockers-ARBs)	"sartan" Candesartan Eprosartan Losartan Irbesartan Telmisartan Valsartan	It blocks the angiotensin II receptor on the surface of the vascular smooth muscle, thereby inhibiting the vasoconstrictive action of Angiotensin II.	Hypertension	Hypotension, fatigue, dizziness, headaches, cough, Upper Respiratory Infection (URI), muscle pain, rhinitis	Use cautiously in patients with renal or heart failure. Please do not use it in pregnancy or breastfeeding.
Hydralazine	Hydralazine	A direct-acting vasodilator that relaxes arteriolar smooth muscle.	Hypertension Hypertensive crisis Preeclampsia Eclampsia CHF	Headaches, dizziness, hypotension, tachycardia, edema, nasal congestion, decreased CBC values.	Take it with food. Please do not use it in pregnancy.
Methyldopa	Methyldopa	It inhibits the vasomotor center, inhibiting sympathetic outflow to the kidneys, heart, and peripheral vasculature.	Hypertension Hypertensive crisis	Sedation, headaches, weakness, dizziness, decreased mental acuity, paresthesia, parkinsonism, choreiform movements, psychic disturbances, nightmares, bradycardia, orthostatic hypotension, nasal congestion, pancreatitis, dry mouth, decreased CBC	Do not give to patients with liver disease or taking MAOIs (antidepressants). Do not use if breastfeeding.

				values, muscle pain, hepatotoxic drug.	

CARDIAC MEDICATIONS					
MEDICATION	EXAMPLES	ACTION	USE	ADVERSE REACTION	RECOMMENDATIONS
Nitroprusside (IV)	Nitroprusside	Relaxes arteriolar and venous smooth muscle.	Hypertensive crisis Reduces preload and afterload shock. Cardiac failure	Headaches, dizziness, loss of consciousness, increased ICP, bradycardia, hypotension, Tachycardia, muscle twitching, diaphoresis, cyanide toxicity, decreased RBCs and WBCs	Keep the patient supine when giving medication. Use cautiously in patients with renal disease, increased ICP, liver disease, acute CHF, hypothyroid, and hyponatremia.
Antilipemic	"statin" Simvastatin Rosuvastatin Pravastatin Atorvastatin Lovastatin Cholestyramine Gemfibrozil		Lower cholesterol	Liver toxicity *Rhabdomyolysis* (muscle pain), Fever, Cough	Give it at the same time every day, usually with the evening meal.

MEAN ARTERIAL PRESSURE

The Mean Arterial Pressure (MAP) is the average pressure in a patient's arteries during one cardiac cycle. MAP between 70 mmHg and 100 mmHg is considered normal. Calculating the

MAP better indicates blood perfusion to vital organs than systolic blood pressure. To calculate the MAP, the nurse can use the following formula:

$$MAP = SBP + 2\,(DBP)/3$$

Example: The patient has a blood pressure of 94 mmHg/54 mmHg.

$$MAP = 94 + 2(54)/3$$

$$MAP = 94 + 108 / 3$$

$$MAP = 202/3$$

$$MAP = 67$$

High MAP

A MAP above 100 mm Hg indicates high blood pressure in the arteries. A patient with a high MAP is at risk of developing clots. If untreated, the heart muscle will be damaged, putting the patient at risk of heart attack, heart failure, and kidney failure.

Low MAP

A MAP below 70 mmHg indicates that essential organs are not receiving the necessary blood to function. If this situation is not addressed, the organs' tissue dies. The damage will be irreversible, putting the patient at risk of stroke or sepsis.

THE MEAN ARTERIAL PRESSURE IS ASSOCIATED WITH BLOOD FLOW AND RESISTANCE. IT INDICATES IF THE PATIENT RECEIVES ENOUGH BLOOD TO SUPPLY ALL MAJOR ORGANS. TOO MUCH RESISTANCE AND PRESSURE WILL IMPEDE THAT FLOW.

(Nall, 2023)

The Ejection Fraction

The ejection fraction measures the heart's ability to pump oxygen-rich blood throughout the body. Blood enters the heart's upper right chamber or the atrium, and during the pause between heartbeats, it passes through a valve into the lower left chamber or left ventricle. Once the ventricle is filled with oxygenated blood, the next heartbeat ejects a quantity of this oxygenated blood out to the body. The standard ejection fraction percentage is 50% to 70%. A higher ejection fraction signifies a healthy and strong heart. When the patient has or is at risk for heart failure, the primary healthcare provider will calculate the ejection fraction.

BECAUSE SOME CHEMOTHERAPY AGENTS HAVE A HIGHER RISK OF BEING CARDIOTOXIC, BEFORE STARTING THE CYCLES, IT IS IMPORTANT TO DETERMINE THE EJECTION FRACTION.

CHAPTER 2 HEMATOLOGY

Hematology is the study, treatment, and prevention of blood-related diseases, vital for overall health. Blood tests offer significant health insights, making this specialty important in various subfields. Hematologists focus on bone marrow, blood coagulation, and severe disorders like anemia and leukemia.

DIAGNOSTIC TESTS

CBC (Complete Blood Count): This test evaluates the cells in the blood and determines patients' overall health. It measures the number, color intensity, and size of red blood cells (RBC), hemoglobin, white cells, and platelets. When the test includes the Differential, it will consist of different mature and immature white blood cells. The differential is essential to assess the immune system cells. This test is usually ordered to rule out anemias (low hemoglobin level), erythrocytosis (high level of red blood cells), leukocytosis (high WBC), leukopenia (low WBC), thrombocytosis (high PLT level), and thrombocytopenia (low PLT level).

WBC (White Blood Count) – The function of the white blood cells is to fight infections. The normal range is 5,000 to 10,000. There are different types of white blood cells with specific functions. White blood cells include neutrophils, lymphocytes, monocytes, eosinophils, and basophils.

Leukocytosis—An increased level of >12,000 white cells is called leukocytosis, an indication of an inflammatory response usually associated with infections. However, it can also indicate the development of bone tumors or hematologic disorders, such as leukemia. This can also occur because of emotional stress, medications, injury, surgery, or excessive exercise.

Nursing Care

Primary nursing care involves assessing the patient for signs and symptoms of infection: discharge or drainage, edema, redness or erythema, and temperature or tenderness. It is essential to monitor the patient's temperature, which is usually ordered to be checked every four hours.

Leukopenia and Neutropenia - Leukopenia is a condition characterized by decreased levels of white cells in blood below the expected values. Most of the white cells are comprised of neutrophils. Neutropenia is an abnormally low level of neutrophils

(<2,000) in blood. Neutrophils are the primary defense against infections. This condition puts the patient at a higher risk for infections.

Nursing Care

Nursing responsibility includes monitoring and protecting the patient from infections, monitoring the temperature (usually ordered every four hours), monitoring diet and visitors, and providing mouth care. Mouth care is essential to prevent stomatitis. Use a soft toothbrush—no fresh flowers or plants. Check the temperature axillary—no uncooked or raw food. Increase protein intake to build the immune system and increase carbohydrates. The diet should be bland and consist of small, frequent meal

Platelets (PLT) - Another name for platelets is thrombocytes. Thrombocytes are clotting cells. Not enough thrombocytes (thrombocytopenia) can be a sign of cancer, and too many can cause a stroke. The standard value or range is 150,000 to 450,000. An abnormal decrease in thrombocyte level (<50,000) in blood puts the patient at risk for bleeding.

Nursing Care

The primary intervention is the prevention of injuries and bleeding. Educating the patient about mouth care, shaving with an electric razor, elimination (stool softener and increased fiber intake), and activities (gentle blowing of the nose and no weightlifting or contact sports) is essential. The bed can be padded and kept in the lowest position. The light in the room should always be on, or a night light can be used. Needle precautions are implemented. A central line might be the best alternative.

Red Blood Cells (RBCs or Erythrocytes)—The primary function of red blood cells is carrying oxygen. Their life cycle is 120 days. The standard value or range is 4.5 to 6.0. A decrease in size and color puts the patient at risk for decreased oxygen levels.

Hemoglobin (Hgb) - Hemoglobin is the iron-rich protein in red blood cells that carries oxygen through the body. If a patient has a condition that interferes with the development of red blood cells, the hemoglobin level will decrease. A low hemoglobin level may be a symptom of cancer or anemia. The standard value or range is 12 to 16 g/dL and varies between men and women.

Hematocrit (HCT) - Hematocrit measures the percentage of red blood cells in the blood and is the best indicator of blood loss. The normal value or range is 38 to 47%.

Nursing Care

Fluid volume-excess = edema. This will result in a lower hematocrit level (hemodilution). The treatment is to administer diuretics.

Fluid-Volume-Deficit=dehydration. This will result in the hematocrit level being higher (hemoconcentration).

Blood cells develop in the bone marrow. If the necessary substances (iron, folic acid, and vitamin B-12) to create new and healthy blood cells are lacking, the blood cells will be defective.

CONDITIONS AND COAGULATION STUDIES

DEEP VEIN THROMBOSIS (DVT) is the development of a clot in a vein, preventing blood from circulating freely throughout the body. Another name is thrombophlebitis. The number one cause is immobility. This may be the result of strict bedrest, MI, CVA, CHF, and obese patients. Signs and symptoms include pain in the dorsiflexion of the foot (Homan's sign). The area might be red and swollen. Treatment includes bedrest, elevation of lower extremity, and warm/moist compresses. The patient will be on anticoagulation medication such as Heparin IV and may continue anticoagulation medication PO, such as Coumadin.

Patient education should be focused on anticoagulation medications and avoid using OTC medications such as aspirin, aspirin-containing medicines and products, steroids, and aminoglycosides.

Partial Thromboplastin Time (PTT) - This test determines how long the blood can clot. The standard value or range is 25 to 38 seconds. The partial thromboplastin time results show why the blood is clotting too fast or too slow by testing the proteins in the blood or coagulation factors. Adding a solution to the blood sample to activate the clotting factors changes the name of the test to activated partial thromboplastin time or aPTT. The test is performed when the patient has a clot to determine why the blood is clotting too fast or too slowly, if the patient had a miscarriage, or if the patient has liver disease. It is also ordered when the patient is receiving a Heparin Drip. If there is an error concerning the administration of Heparin, the Heparin antidote is Protamine Sulfate IV. The goal for a patient on a Heparin rip is up to 70. The bleed-out zone is >100.

Prothrombin Time (PT)—The prothrombin time is ordered to determine why the blood is clotting too fast. The standard value or range is 11 to 15 seconds. This test is also ordered when the patient takes the anticoagulation medication or blood thinner Coumadin. If the patient is on Coumadin, the PT is measured using a calculation measurement called the International Normalized Ratio (INR).

International Normalized Ratio (INR)—This blood test monitors the use of Coumadin. The standard value or range for INR is 2 to 3 seconds, the therapeutic level of Coumadin. Coumadin's antidote is Vitamin K. Green leafy vegetables and raisins are rich in vitamin K. However, foods and herbal medicines can increase or decrease the PT/INR and PTT levels, and it is essential to educate the patient.

Herbal Medicines that Increase PT/INR, PTT	
Medication	Action
Bilberry	Decreases blood sugar and triglycerides. It can make the patient anemic or jaundiced.

Black Cohosh	They are used for PMS and menopause. Please do not use it for more than six months.
Capsicum	It controls pain and is used for chronic pain, rheumatoid arthritis, or shingles. It causes diarrhea, mouth sores, and bronchospasm. Please do not give it to patients receiving ACE inhibitors. Cocaine and capsicum together cause death.
Chamomile	
Feverfew	Used to induce labor.
Echinacea	It fights viruses and shortens the length of colds. It should be taken at most 14 days.
Evening Primrose	Used to induce labor. Dilates the cervix.
Garlic	It stabilizes blood pressure, protects the heart, increases HDL, and keeps blood sugar and blood pressure low. It also protects against gastric cancer and stroke.
Ginger	Antiemetic (morning/movement sickness). Too much ginger causes arrhythmia.
Gingko	It increases blood flow to the brain and circulation in the legs. Please only use it for up to three months.

Herbal Medicines that Decrease PT/INR, PTT	
Medication	Action
St. John's Wort	They are used for depression. It damages sperm and causes infertility. When used with MAOI (Monoamine oxidase inhibitors), blood pressure decreases. MAOIs are antidepression medications.
Green Tea	Blocks iron absorption.
Nettle	Used to lose weight. It is a natural diuretic.
Ginseng	Boosts concentration. It has estrogen-like effects. Use at most three months.

Bone Marrow Biopsy/Aspiration—This painful procedure is performed on patients with a low CBC and is usually performed under moderate sedation at the bedside.

Nursing Care – Make sure the patient has received education regarding the procedure and has a signed consent form. During the procedure, the nurse should focus on the amount of medication administered. Maintain the patient at least 2L of O2 via nasal cannula unless the physician orders a different amount and monitors the blood pressure. This procedure is excruciating, and the physician should administer numbing medication at the site. Occasionally, and depending on the person performing the procedure, taking the blood and bone samples may be challenging. The nurse should act as the patient's advocate if the procedure is being performed too often and the patient is in pain and uncomfortable.

Offer information on how to care for the site after the procedure. It is essential to offer support and listen to patient and family concerns. Iron intake stimulates the bone marrow (red meat, egg yolks, and liver). Milk blocks iron from being absorbed.

HEMATOLOGIC DISORDERS AND CONDITIONS

ANEMIAS

Anemia is a deficiency of red blood cells. It can be caused by an abnormal or decreased production of healthy red blood cells or by acute or long-term blood loss or breakdown of red blood cells, called hemolysis. There are different types of anemia. Symptoms include fatigue, weakness, and shortness of breath.

Hemolytic Anemia is caused by an abnormal breakdown (hemolysis) of red blood cells (erythrocytes).

Iron Deficiency Anemia is the most common anemia. It is caused by not eating iron-rich food or losing too much blood from an injury or a disease. Signs and symptoms include pallor, fatigue (due to low iron level), vertigo, weakness, the patient always being cold, and dizziness.

Nursing Care

The patient is at high risk for falls, so protecting the patient from injuries is essential. The diet should be high in iron, with increased fluids and fiber to prevent constipation. Iron supplements should be taken on an empty stomach before meals. Ambulation will help absorb the iron.

Pernicious Anemia—Pernicious anemia is a hematologic condition caused by a vitamin B-12 deficiency. It is an autoimmune condition that prevents the body from absorbing vitamin B-12. It is more frequent in patients with gastric surgery and cancer. Signs and symptoms include paresthesia (numbness and tingling signifying neurological damage), red tongue, and stomatitis. The patient will be sent for a gastric analysis and a Schilling's 24-hour urine test. A positive test will show no B-12 in the urine.

Nursing Care

The patient is prone to injury, and nursing's goal is to prevent further neurological damage. As a safety measure, a skin assessment is essential. The patient will receive vitamin B-12 for life, and the diet should be regular and well-balanced.

Aplastic Anemia – This condition develops when the stem cells in the bone marrow do not produce enough blood cells. It also results from underdevelopment (hypoplasia) or aplasia (loss of function). It is more common in patients who frequently use NSAIDs, such as Ibuprofen, in cancer patients receiving chemotherapy, and in people who have been exposed to chemical toxins. Signs and symptoms include low RBs, WBCs, and low PLTs, as well as signs of very unhealthy bone marrow. The patient will need a Bone Marrow Transplant (the only cure).

Nursing Care

The patient is at high risk for injury, infection, and bleeding. The primary nursing intervention is to implement safety interventions to prevent injuries. Follow the care that must be offered for the cell deficiencies indicated above.

INHERITED ANEMIAS

Sickle-Cell Disorder – An inherited disorder affecting the red blood cells' shape, turning round, flexible discs into "C" shape, stiff, and sticky cells that block blood flow. The patient suffers from unbearable pain.

Thalassemia—In this condition, the body produces less hemoglobin, resulting in small red blood cells and anemia.

Nursing Care

The patient must consent before administering blood, which is suitable for 24 hours. Have a 0.9% Normal Saline (NS) available. The nurse must verify that all the information on the bag is the same as that found on the blood transfusion document obtained from the lab when the transfusion is handed over to the nurse. Errors related to the administration of the wrong blood type have death or life consequences. Obtain baseline vital signs and monitor the patient throughout the administration process. Be ready of intervene if a blood transfusion reaction occurs.

Anemias are treated with Blood Transfusion. Blood transfusions replace volume, oxygen, fluid, and clotting factors.

ANEMIAS				
Condition	Cause	Presentation	Signs and Symptoms	Treatment
Iron-deficiency Anemia	Hemoglobin synthesis is impaired. RBCs are smaller.	Low iron level in the body		Cause and iron supplements
Hemolytic Anemia	Disease-causing hemolysis. Congenital or acquired.	Abnormal breakdown of RBCs.	Jaundice, enlarged spleen, and liver.	Cause
Aplastic Anemia	Bone marrow failure	Hypoplasia or Aplasia. Inadequate number of RBCs, WBCs, and PLTs	Fever, bruises on the skin and mucous membranes.	Cause and severity
Pernicious Anemia	Autoimmune. Inability to absorb vitamin B-12	Low B-112 levels	Paresthesia, red tongue, and stomatitis.	Cause and Vitamin B-12

Polycythemia Vera (also known as *Myeloproliferative neoplasm*)	Gene mutation causes a problem with blood cell production. It is rare, but it is more common in male adults between 50 and 75.	Enlarged spleen. The bone marrow makes too many RBCs. Complication: Blood Clots	Itchy skin, numbness, and tingling in hands, feet, arms, and legs. Bloating and abdominal pain. Unusual bleeding. Swelling and pain of the big toe. Shortness of breath and Dyspnea. Bone pain.	Frequent blood draws. Aspirin. Antihistamine for itching.
Sickle Cell Anemia/Disorder	Inherited.	RBCs have "C" shape. Cells are rigid and sticky.	Severe episodes of pain. Swollen hands and feet. Frequent infections and visual problems. Delayed growth.	Symptoms
Thalassemia	DNA mutation. Inherited.	Low hemoglobin. RBCs destruction.	Weakness or fatigue. Slow growth. Jaundice. Pale appearance. Deformities in facial bones. Dark urine and abdominal swelling.	Frequent blood transfusions. Bone marrow transplants. *Iron chelation therapy* (removal of heavy metals from the body).

Polycythemia Vera is characterized by a blood sample with too many RBCs. The HCT and Hgb are elevated. Patients will present hypertension (HTN) and Congestive Heart Failure (CHF), which puts them at an increased risk for clots.

Nursing Care

The number one intervention is to assess patients for clotting. Patients will receive IV fluids to dilute the blood and be required to donate blood frequently. Check HCT every two weeks.

CLOTTING DISORDERS

Disseminated Intravascular Coagulation (DIC) – Widespread clotting deficiency occurs within the blood vessels, meaning there are no clotting factors in the circulation going to the microcirculation. This might be caused by trauma related to surgery. It is often seen in patients with cancer, sepsis, or pancreatitis. Petechia is a sign of a complication and indicates a problem with bleeding.

Nursing Care

Blood laboratories include PLTs, PT, and fibrinogen (a coagulation factor). The patient will receive cryoprecipitate transfusion and IV fluids. Cryoprecipitates take factor VIII back into the circulation.

CRYOPRECIPITATE IS A BLOOD PRODUCT OBTAINED FROM THE PLASMA , RICH IN SPECIFIC INSOLUBLE BLOOD PROTEINS (COAGULATION FACTORS) PLAYING AN IMPORTANT ROLE IN MANAGING BOTH THE CLOTTING AND CLOT-DISSOLVING PROCESSES.

BLOOD TRANSFUSION

The main components of blood are red blood cells, white blood cells, platelets, and plasma. Whole blood is 55% plasma and 45% blood cells. Blood transfusion is the intravenous administration of blood and blood products. Blood can be donated by another person or by the patient. The patient's blood is stored and used when needed.

Blood Types

The absence or presence of specific antigens and antibodies categorizes the four major blood groups, creating eight blood types: O+, O-, A+, A-, B+, B-, AB+, and AB-. The ABO system consists of A and B antigens. A person with A antigen produces type A blood. B antigen produces type B blood. Having A and B antigens produces type AB blood. Not having antigens leads to type O blood. People with type O- are considered universal donors for red blood cells. People who have type AB+ are considered universal recipients. O+ is the most common blood type. AB- is the rarest blood type.

Antibodies are developed around six months old. Type A blood has anti-B antibodies, Type B blood has anti-A antibodies, and Type AB does not have antibodies. Type O has anti-A and anti-B antibodies.

Blood type is inherited. The Rh+ factor indicates that the blood type has the D antigen, while the Rh- factor indicates that the blood type does not have the D antigen. This is important for blood transfusions and pregnancies. The administration of the wrong Rh factor will cause the patient to develop a hemolytic reaction. Receiving the wrong blood type will trigger the immune system to reject the blood and attack the blood that has been transfused. Some complications of blood transfusions include allergic reactions, an immune hemolytic reaction, or blood-borne infections. A person who develops an allergic reaction will experience symptoms like hives and itching that can be treated with antihistamines. A hemolytic response is a more serious condition that usually occurs when the person receives the wrong blood type. If the person develops a hemolytic reaction, the immune system will release a substance that will damage the kidneys, presenting signs and symptoms such as fever, back and flank pain, and red or brown urine.

Parent 1 Blood Type	O	O	O	O	A	A	A	B	B	AB
Parent 2 Blood Type	O	A	B	AB	A	B	AB	B	AB	AB
O	✓	✓	✓		✓	✓		✓		

Possible Blood Type of the Child	A		✓	✓	✓	✓	✓	✓		✓	✓
	B				✓		✓	✓	✓	✓	✓
	AB						✓	✓		✓	✓

Before a transfusion, the blood undergoes tests for potential infections, viruses, and bacteria. Although a patient can develop an illness or disease, the chance of developing an infection after a blood transfusion, such as HIV, Hepatitis B or C, or the West Nile Virus, is very low.

A PERSON WITH AN O-NEGATIVE BLOOD TYPE IS CONSIDERED A UNIVERSAL DONOR.

Blood Type	Blood Type Compatibility
A+	A+, A-, O+, O-
A-	A-, O-
B+	B+, B-, O+, O-
B-	B-, O-
AB+	Universal Recipient
AB-	AB-, A-, B-, O-
O+	O+, O-
O-	Universal Donor

The nurse is responsible for reviewing the blood thoroughly to prevent complications for the patient. When the patient has an order to administer whole blood or any other blood product, the nurse must follow the healthcare facility protocols for blood transfusion. Appropriate time administration must be followed depending on the blood product being transfused. Retrieval of blood from the blood bank should not be delegated to unlicensed clinical personnel. Information on the blood bag must be reviewed with two nurses. The patient's condition should be monitored throughout the blood transfusion.

CHAPTER 3

ONCOLOGY

Oncology studies the abnormal proliferation of abnormal cells in the body, known as cancer. Abnormal cells multiply uncontrollably, interrupting the cell's normal lifecycle and function. They interact and are used throughout the body. Oncology affects how body system operate and communicate, interrupting metabolism and homeostasis. It specializes in the diagnosis and treatment of cancer.

CANCER

The uncontrollable proliferation of those abnormal and damaged cells. Those cells stay together, forming a cluster of damaged cells or tumors. Tumors can be benign or malignant. Benign tumors do not spread and, after being removed, do not grow back. Malignant tumors invade organs, interrupting their function. Cancer tumors create their circulatory system. They can be solid or not, such as blood cancers, and are described by the type of cell that formed them.

Staging	Survival
I – One node	100%
II – Two or more nodes on the same side of the diaphragm	98%
III – Widespread lymphatic system involvement showing nodes on both sides of the diaphragm	50%
IV – Extra lymphatic involvement	0%

RISK FACTORS

RISK FACTORS FOR CANCER	
Cancer Type	Risk Factors
Breast Cancer	Older than 50 years old Family History Menarche before 12 years old, Menopause after 55 years old Pregnancy after 35 years old, Nulliparity
Cervical Cancer	Sexually transmitted infections Sexual activity before 17 years, Multiple sex partners Smoking
Endometrial/Uterine Cancer	Postmenopausal women

	Obesity and late menopause Nulliparity, Infertility, Irregular menarche History of breast or ovarian cancer Prolonged use of unopposed estrogen treatment
Ovarian Cancer	Family history of cancer: ovarian, breast, colon Nulliparity: Pregnancy after 35 years Early menarche, Late menopause
Colon Cancer	Dietary factor dominant, Increased dietary fat, Alcohol. Genetic Ulcerative colitis, Chron's Disease, Familial polyposis (genetics)
Prostate Cancer	Genetics Above 50 years High-fat diet
Stomach Cancer	Family history of gastric cancer Pernicious anemia Helicobacter Pylori Infection, Chronic gastritis, Benign Peptic ulcer disease Rubber or Coal worker
Skin Cancer	Exposure to sun, easily sunburned. Ultraviolet radiation, ionizing radiation, changing moles.
Laryngeal Cancer	Tobacco, alcohol, Smoking Fumes, Radiation COPD Excessive use of voice
Bladder Cancer	Exposure to chemicals Smoking

Testicular Cancer	Undescended testicles (*Cryptorchidism)*

CARCINOMAS

The most common cancer, carcinomas, are formed from epithelial cells. *Adenocarcinomas* are formed from glandular tissue, which are cells that produce fluids. Glandular tissue includes cells that produce fluids. Cancers include breast, colon, and prostate cancer. *Basal Cell Carcinomas* are formed in the epidermis's base (basal) layer. *Squamous Cell Carcinomas* are the cells that line organs such as the stomach, intestines, lungs, bladder, and kidneys.

Breast Cancer

The risk factor is a history of the maternal side of the family with breast cancer and a sister or relative with ovarian cancer. Thirty-five-year-old primigravida is at most risk for breast cancer. Early menses and late menopause are risks of breast cancer. Signs and symptoms of breast cancer include a mass in the breast that may be palpable or non-palpable. Breast cancer is diagnosed through mammography and biopsy. The treatment varies depending on the extension of the tumor and stage.

Lumpectomy (removal of the mass), modified mastectomy (removal of the minor pectoral muscles), and double mastectomy. Patients will undergo chemotherapy and radiation therapy. Depending on the extension of the cancer cells in the system, the patient may receive chemotherapy as part of the treatment. Most of the patients are put on a *PO medication* for five years that will prevent estrogen from binding in tissues with an increased number of estrogen receptors (uterus, breast, vagina, and ovaries). Adverse reactions include weight gain or loss, fluid retention, anemia, retinopathy, hepatic necrosis, osteoporosis, and risk for uterine cancer. Increases Coumadin effect and should not be given within two hours of receiving antacids.

Nursing Care

Before surgery, Teach the patient how to TCDB (turn, cough, deep breath). Teach the patient also to do wall-walking exercises and hand exercises. *After surgery,* educate the patient to keep the arm elevated for 24 hours and assess circulation and how the patient is coping. A mastectomy alters a person's body image. Teach the patient how to care for the affected arm and observe signs and symptoms of *lymphedema* (cellular waste accumulates in the area after removing lymph nodes) and infection.

Cervical Cancer

The main risk factors for the development of cervical cancer are multiple sex partners, chronic cervical infection, human papillomavirus (HPV), and smoking. Smoking is a risk factor for bladder, oral, cervical, esophageal, lung, and laryngeal cancers (BOCELL). The human papillomavirus (HPV) can attack different parts of the body. One distinctive sign is the development of warts. These can appear on hands, feet, and other areas. When the virus attacks the genitals, it is a sexually transmitted disease. The patient may not experience any symptoms of HPV.

Ovarian Cancer

Risk factors include infertility, nulliparity, and breast cancer.

The treatment for these cancers includes chemotherapy, surgery, and radiation. One of the main chemotherapeutic agents used for ovarian and advanced breast cancer is *Taxol,* usually used with *Doxorubicin (Adriamycin*). The main adverse reactions are hypotension, bradycardia, anemia, peripheral neuropathy, alopecia, increased liver enzymes, and triglycerides.

LEUKEMIAS

Leukemias are cancers formed from the bone marrow and are not solid tumors. These cancers are abnormal white blood cells that form in the bone marrow, reducing the number of healthy blood cells. This results in decreased oxygen levels in the tissues and difficulty for the body in fighting infections and controlling bleeding.

LYMPHOMAS

Lymphomas are cancers that begin in lymphocytes, which are T and B cells. These cancers disrupt the disease-fighting ability of white blood cells.

Hodgkin's Lymphoma

Cancer of the lymphatic system. It is known as a “young person’s cancer” because it is more common in 20-year-old people. It is also common in people >50. There is a familial risk. Cells are formed from B cells.

Signs and Symptoms

Lymph node enlargement that is fixed and painless, night sweats, temperature > 100.4, weight loss, and 20% pain at the site after alcohol intake. The patient undergoes a biopsy. The presentation of Reed-Sternberg cancer cells will give a positive result for the biopsy.

Non-Hodgkin’s Lymphoma

Widespread lymphatic tissue tumor that presents regular lymphatic cells. These lymphoma cells are formed from T or B cells and can grow slowly or quickly. Treatment is the administration of chemotherapy, antibiotics, and medication to increase WBC, PLT, HGB, and HCT. The patient may receive blood transfusion, albumin, and antibodies.

Multiple Myeloma (MM)

This is bone cancer, presenting plasma cell tumors that destroy the bone marrow. These cells develop tumors all over the body.

Signs and Symptoms

Patients experience pain, fractures, high calcium levels in the blood, low RBCs (anemia), low WBCs (infections), low PLTs (bleeding), and Bence-Jones proteinuria test. It is not normal for patients to have protein in their urine. When the doctor suspects that the patient has MM will order this test. This is shown only in patients with bone cancer. The patient is at risk of developing Gout. The calcium removed from the bone puts the patient at risk for kidney stones.

Nursing Care

The priority of care is pain management. Nursing must provide comfort, increase fluid intake, encourage ambulation, and provide safety measures.

MELANOMAS

This type of cancer is formed from the specialized cells that give skin its color, melanin. They usually form on the skin but can also form in the eyes.

BRAIN AND SPINAL CORD TUMORS

Tumors related to the brain and the spinal cord are named according to the cells in which they are formed and the area in the nervous system.

SARCOMAS

Sarcomas form in bone and soft tissues, such as muscle, fat, blood, lymph vessels, tendons, and ligaments. Osteosarcomas, including Kaposi sarcoma, are cancers of the bone.

CANCER TREATMENTS

Chemotherapy involves administering drugs that use chemicals to kill fast-growing abnormal cells, interrupting the body's homeostasis. Chemotherapy is used for other conditions other than cancers. For example, bone marrow diseases and immune system conditions are often treated with the use of chemotherapeutic medications. In recent years, it has also been used to treat other conditions, such as Multiple Sclerosis (MS), Chron's Disease (CD), and Rheumatoid Arthritis (RA). Drugs are administered alone or in combination with multiple medications. Different ways chemotherapy is administered are IV infusions, pills, shots, and creams, and administered directly into one area of the body or directly to the cancer tumor. This therapy is very aggressive, identifying and destroying cancer cells and, unfortunately, also good cells. Chemotherapy cycles may last at least six months. Although chemotherapy is effective, the side effects range from mild to severe. Mild side effects are treatable. Other side effects cause serious complications. Cancer patients who receive chemotherapy agents will become immunocompromised because these medications will affect the bone marrow, decreasing the number of white cells created, especially neutrophils.

Side effects of chemotherapeutic drugs include nausea, vomiting, diarrhea, constipation, pain, hair loss, loss of appetite, fatigue, fever, mouth sores, easy bruising, and bleeding. These symptoms become evident after months or years of treatment. Those include infertility, damage to lung tissue, kidney problems, heart problems, and nerve damage (peripheral neuropathy). There is always a risk for the development of other cancers.

Nursing Care

Patient education should include the importance of personal hygiene and caution in public and crowded places. Patients should use extra caution if they have pets. Avoid unpasteurized foods and be cautious when handling and cooking meats, moldy cheeses, and fresh produce.

Radiotherapy is administered externally or internally. External is the most common type. In this type, the beams of high-energy radiation are directed toward the tumor, avoiding healthy tissue. Internal radiation, also called *brachytherapy*, is given by inserting a solid radioactive "seed" inside or close to the cancer tumor. This "seed" continuously releases radiation for an extended period. Another way to administer internal radiation is by vein, which is called *radioimmunotherapy.* It can also be administered in liquid form.

Radiation side effects include fatigue, nausea, vomiting, diarrhea, and headaches. Additional side effects are dry, itchy scalp, hair loss, mouth sores, urinary frequency, swallowing pain, abdominal bloating or cramps, and decreased appetite. Nurses pay close attention to skin irritation and burning sensations the patients complain of, such as a burning feeling in their throat or chest and pain or a burning sensation when they pee. As with chemotherapy, some side effects will appear after several weeks. There is also the risk of developing other cancers in the future.

Surgery removes cancer tumors from the body in several ways. Cryosurgery, which uses extreme cold to destroy abnormal tissue, is often used in early-stage skin cancer. Lasers, beams of light used to cut tissue, are also used to remove, shrink, or destroy cancer tumors. Hyperthermia exposes the cancer cells to high temperatures, damaging or destroying them. *Photodynamic Therapy* is a treatment where medications that react to light are administered, activating the drugs and killing the cancer cells.

The main side effects of surgery are pain and infection. Nurses must assess the pain level and continue to manage it accordingly. If the patient presents signs of infection, notify the physician of the possibility of the development of internal infection. If the wound is visible, evaluate it for signs and symptoms of infection.

CHAPTER 4 THE RESPIRATORY SYSTEM

The respiratory system, an intricate network that includes the lungs, and airways such as the trachea, bronchi, and bronchioles, along with the diaphragm, larynx, pharynx, nose, and mouth, is vital for life. Its primary role is to facilitate the inhalation of oxygen and the exhalation of carbon dioxide. Beyond this essential function, it plays a critical role in maintaining homeostasis and defending the body against harmful particles and pathogens, while also

DIAGNOSTIC TESTS AND PROCEDURES

Bronchoscopy

This procedure is used to diagnose or treat a patient with respiratory symptoms related to a possible disease. Consent should be obtained before scheduling the procedure. The patient should be NPO because moderate sedation with Versed is given. Patients will also receive localized sedation with Lidocaine. Patient education is related to being unable to speak while the scope is in the throat. After the procedure, the gag reflex will be assessed, and the patient will remain NPO until the gag reflex returns.

Sputum Specimen

This test is used to diagnose disease. A sputum specimen should be obtained before starting antibiotic medication. It is received early in the morning, and the mouth should be rinsed with water only. The patient will breathe a deep breath three times and then cough sputum into a sterile container.

Pulmonary Function Test (PFT)

This test assesses lung volume and capacity to determine how well the lungs work and exchange air. It diagnoses COPD, pulmonary fibrosis, and asthma and is also used before thoracic surgery. Different types of breathing tests are included to assess lung function. The physician will order this test if the patient has symptoms that suggest the lung function or airway is compromised. Some symptoms include coughing that produces mucus, difficulty breathing and dyspnea, wheezing, complaints of pain and pressure while breathing, and chest tightness. The patient should avoid caffeine and be NPO. The test requires recording the patient's personal information, such as height and weight, age, sex, and race.

Spirometry

Spirometry is the most common PFT. It measures *vital capacity.* Vital Capacity is the maximum exhalation possible after maximum inhalation. This will decrease in COPD patients. *Tidal Volume* is the amount of air inhaled and exhaled while breathing. *Inspiratory Reserve Volume* is the maximum amount of air a person can inhale after a normal inhalation. *Expiratory Reserve Volume* is the maximum amount of air exhaled after normal exhalation. Exhalation is decreased in COPD patients. *Dead Space* is the air that is not exchanged -the Dead Space increases in COPD patients.

Thoracentesis

This procedure removes fluid or gas from the pleural space of the lung. The pleural space has a lubricant that facilitates lung expansion. If additional fluid builds in the space, it will compress the lungs, making it difficult for them to function well. This is called pleural effusion. The patient sits up with arms extended over the table. A needle is placed into the pleural space to drain the extra fluid. Nurses monitor vital signs, especially BP. Hypovolemia and pneumothorax are the main risks of this procedure. Other risks include infection and liver or spleen injury, which are rare.

Pneumothorax

Pneumothorax is an air or fluid found in the pleural space of the lung. It is diagnosed through chest X-rays, and ABGs present respiratory acidosis. To treat a patient with pneumothorax, a thoracentesis is performed, and a *chest tube* is placed. This is connected to a closed drainage system that removes the fluids accumulated in the pleural space. The patient should be kept in a low semi-fowler's position. The closed drainage system should be placed lower than the patient. Signs and symptoms of pneumothorax are sudden sharp chest pain with *dyspnea* (difficulty breathing) and possibly shock. During auscultation, breath will be absent sounds over the area, asymmetry of chest movement with breathing, and tracheal deviation towards the unaffected side.

V/Q Scan

A Ventilation/Perfusion Scan is a two-part test to diagnose a lung blood clot known as *pulmonary embolism* or PE. It measures the airflow (ventilation) and the blood flow (perfusion) in the lungs. In this test, the patient receives an IV radioactive dye. Then, the scanning is performed to assess the blood perfusion. Then, the patient breathes radioactive gas. Then, scanning is performed to determine the ventilation. Before the test, allergies to dye are assessed. After the test, the patient must increase fluid intake to flush out the radioactive dye.

Oxygen Administration

Low-flow oxygen administration is room air mixed with oxygen administered through a nasal cannula except ~~via~~ when using a Venturi Mask. High-flow oxygen administration delivers precise amounts of oxygen using the Venturi mask. A humidifier (bubbler) is recommended to prevent dryness of the mucous membranes in the nose. When a patient uses a nasal canula, it is essential to assess ears, nares, and prongs. A mask should be cleaned at least every two hours. The patient's face should be wiped.

CONDITIONS

ASTHMA

This condition is characterized by bronchial constriction or spasms that prevent air exhalation. Irritants, cold air, or allergens cause this condition. The patient is treated with an albuterol nebulizer, steroids, Aminophylline, and Theophylline IV. It is essential to assess the BP because the patient is at risk of hypotension. When a patient's asthma exacerbates, stay calm and stay with the patient.

CHRONIC OBSTRUCTIVE PULMONARY DISEASE (COPD)

Irreversible airflow obstruction is associated with an inflammatory response in the lungs, acute bronchitis, and emphysema. Asthma is not associated with COPD; however, COPD patients may have a history of asthma. Signs and Symptoms include wheezing, dyspnea, cyanosis, fever, tachypnea, barrel chest, orthopnea, altered mental status, and elevated jugular venous pressure (JVP).

CHRONIC BRONCHITIS

Chronic productive cough that lasts over three months for two consecutive years or more. This condition is caused by irritation and inflammation in the lining of the bronchi caused by a virus such as influenza. In chronic bronchitis, the patient develops increased phlegm, making it difficult to exchange gases. A distinctive symptom is chest pain that feels more like soreness. The patient will also experience fever and fatigue.

EMPHYSEMA

Emphysema is the overdistension of alveolar spaces causing air-trapping, barrel chest, and impaired oxygen and carbon dioxide (CO_2) gas exchange. The patient develops *respiratory acidosis*. When the patient has a low oxygen level in ABGs is driven to breathe. COPD patients should not receive more than 2L O_2 via NC, or patients will become oxygen dependent. Treatment includes an albuterol nebulizer and inhaler, steroid inhaler, exacerbation antibiotics, and expectorants (Guaifenesin, Robitussin, etc.). Take a bronchodilator inhaler before a steroid inhaler. Rinse mouth well after. MDI – hold the inhaler 1-2 inches (max 5cm) from the mouth.

Nursing Care

Push fluids, encourage bedrest to conserve oxygen, improve oral hygiene, and intake small, frequent high-protein/high-calorie diets for energy. Educate on smoking cessation, pursed-lip breathing, and postural drainage (position patient so gravity helps mobilize secretions while clapping and vibrating on chest). Additional education includes avoiding colds and smoking, remaining in a humid environment, resting, and staying on schedule for flu and pneumonia vaccines. Patients diagnosed with COPD cannot receive more than 3 to 4L of oxygen.

EMBOLISM

Pulmonary Embolism

The patient suddenly complains of dyspnea and chest pain. Nurse intervention includes placing the patient in a high Fowler's position, administering oxygen, and getting help. Treatment involves the administration of blood thinners, clot removal, and vein filter placement.

Air Embolism

This can occur during central IV cap or line change. The patient will experience the same symptoms as above. The nurse places the patient in the left lateral position with the head lower than the body. This position helps to increase blood flow to the heart and facilitates breathing. Get help.

PNEUMONIA

The alveolar spaces fill with exudate and inflammatory cells, causing lung consolidation and affecting the functional tissue. Lung consolidation is caused by pus, blood, or fluid that replaces the air in the lung. When an x-ray is performed, the lung will look solid versus air-filled. Caused by bacteria and viruses, the alveoli or air sacs cannot perform gas exchange. It is diagnosed with chest X-rays, sputum cultures (C&S), and ABGs. The patient will present respiratory acidosis. The treatment includes antibiotics, oxygen administration, Tylenol for fever, and the use of a nebulizer. The nurse places the patient in a high Fowler's position and increases fluid intake.

Thoracic Surgery

Pneumonectomy	Lobectomy
Removal of the lung	Removal of the lobe of the lung
The nurse places the patient on the operative side, supports the chest while coughing, and encourages arm exercises on the affected side to prevent contracture. The nurse also provides pain medication every 30 minutes before deep-breathing and coughing exercises and supports the incision.	The nurse places the patient on the unaffected side to allow affected lung expansion.

Aspiration Pneumonia

This condition is caused by the aspiration of foreign substances through the respiratory system into the lungs. These can be food, drinks, or saliva. Patients who have poor gag reflex or dysphagia (difficulty swallowing) after a stroke or trauma are at risk of developing this condition. Other risk factors include general anesthesia, multiple sclerosis, myasthenia gravis, gastroesophageal reflux disease (GERD), and the insertion of tubes for diagnostic purposes or treatment.

In a normal situation, the epiglottis in the trachea's upper opening prevents foreign objects from entering the lungs. Aspiration is an emergency.

HISTOPLASMOSIS

This is a fungal lung infection caused by inhaling spores in the droppings (feces) of birds, bats, and cats. The signs and symptoms include late-night fever, sweat, and cough. It looks like TB. It is diagnosed by sputum culture (C&S), open lung biopsy, and chest x-ray. The treatment is *amphotericin B* IV, and antifungal medication. Before administering this medication, the patient should be pre-medicated with Tylenol to prevent increased temperature. The nurse assesses the IV site for *phlebitis* and monitors I&O, potassium, BUN, Creatinine, and CBC levels.

Education includes avoidance of caves and wet droppings of birds before shoveling or removing them.

PLEURAL EFFUSION

This is the abnormal accumulation of fluid in the pleural space caused by an imbalance in the pressure and drainage of the lymphatic fluid. This is necessary for the correct functioning of the lungs. This occurs in patients diagnosed with CHF and cirrhosis or patients receiving peritoneal dialysis (PD). This imbalance can also occur due to cancer, pulmonary embolism, pancreatitis, or medications. Diagnosis will be followed by performing a thoracentesis and thoracostomy (chest.)

PNEUMOTHORAX

This is an abnormal presence of air in the space between the parietal and visceral pleurae, known as the pleural cavity. There are two types of pneumothoraxes: spontaneous, traumatic, or tension.

Spontaneous Pneumothorax is classified as primary and secondary. Primary spontaneous pneumothorax develops in patients with no history of lung disease. Secondary spontaneous pneumothorax happens in patients with underlying lung diseases, such as COPD, TB, or asthma.

Traumatic Pneumothorax develops because of a traumatic event, such as a car accident, gunshot wound, or stab wound. It can also be the result of a needle biopsy, thoracentesis, or chest surgery.

Tension Pneumothorax is diagnosed when air is trapped in the pleural space resulting from any condition or procedure mentioned for spontaneous or traumatic pneumothorax. When the air is trapped, the mediastinum cavity shifts or moves toward the unaffected lung, causing depression in the diaphragm on the side of the affected lung.

Signs and symptoms include chest pain, dyspnea, cyanosis, tachycardia, adventitious breath sounds, jugular venous distention, tracheal deviation (on tension pneumothorax), and hypotension. Treatments include oxygen administration, a thoracostomy tube (chest tube) placement, or needle aspiration.

LARYNGEAL CANCER

The patient will complain of pain in the throat when taking hot citrus or carbonated liquids. The main risk factor is smoking.

Laryngectomy

This is the removal of the larynx (voice box), usually related to cancer. The number one cause is smoking. Before the procedure, establishing an alternative means of communication with the patient is essential. Nursing diagnosis included altered body image and altered communication. Education is like the one offered to tracheostomy patients. Apply suction intermittently for over 10 seconds while rotating and removing the suction catheter. Have the patient take five quick breaths before suctioning. No swimming. Humidify the environment and wear the filter over the opening to prevent dust from entering the airway. Avoid cold. One important consideration is having smoke alarms in the home because the patient loses the sense of smell.

LUNG CANCER

Risk factors are smoking, passive secondhand smoking, environmental and occupational exposures (asbestos), genetic predisposition, COPD, and TB.

TUBERCULOSIS (TB)

This condition remains one of the world's leading infectious disease killers (CDC, 2024). Despite being treatable and curable, TB incidence has increased in the United States. It is caused by a bacterium, Mycobacterium Tuberculosis, transmitted through droplets suspended in the air. Symptoms include fatigue, fever and chills, night sweats, coughing, and hemoptysis (coughing up blood). There are two types of TB.

Latent TB

In this condition, the patient carries the disease without presenting symptoms or infecting others.

TB Disease

The person diagnosed with the disease has symptoms and is highly contagious. Immunocompromised patients, such as cancer and HIV/AIDS patients, are more likely to get this disease.

When a person starts treatment but does not complete it, the disease becomes Multidrug-Resistant TB. The bacteria remain in the body and become more difficult to treat and destroy.

PULMONARY EDEMA

This is inflammation that occurs when a person experiences direct trauma to the lungs. The alveoli (where gas exchange occurs) become filled with fluid, making gas exchange difficult. Signs and symptoms include wheezing, hypoxia, headache, cyanosis, anxiety, cough, and altered mental status. Diagnosis is done through chest x-ray, ABG test, echocardiogram, and pulmonary artery catheterization. The patient will receive oxygen therapy, intubation, and morphine administration or a hyperbaric oxygen chamber.

ARTERIAL BLOOD GASES (ABGs)

This blood test measures oxygen in arterial blood and identifies acid-base imbalances. It helps identify conditions that affect the respiratory and circulatory systems. The respiratory therapist draws ABGs after first assessing the radial artery. The blood should be drawn from the artery, not a vein. The arterial blood gases test measures the amount of oxygen and hemoglobin in the blood, oxygen saturation in the body, the pressure of oxygen dissolved in the blood, how well oxygen moves throughout the body, how well carbon dioxide is removed from the body, and the blood pH. They apply pressure to the site for five minutes. The specimen is placed in ice to prevent O2 release.

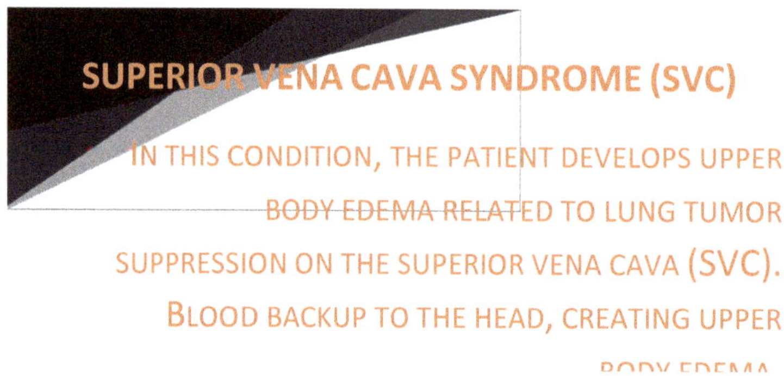

ARTERIAL BLOOD GASES

Normal Values	
pH	7.35 - 7.45
pCO2 (acid)	35 - 45
HCO3 (alkaline; base)	22 - 26
pO2	80 - 100

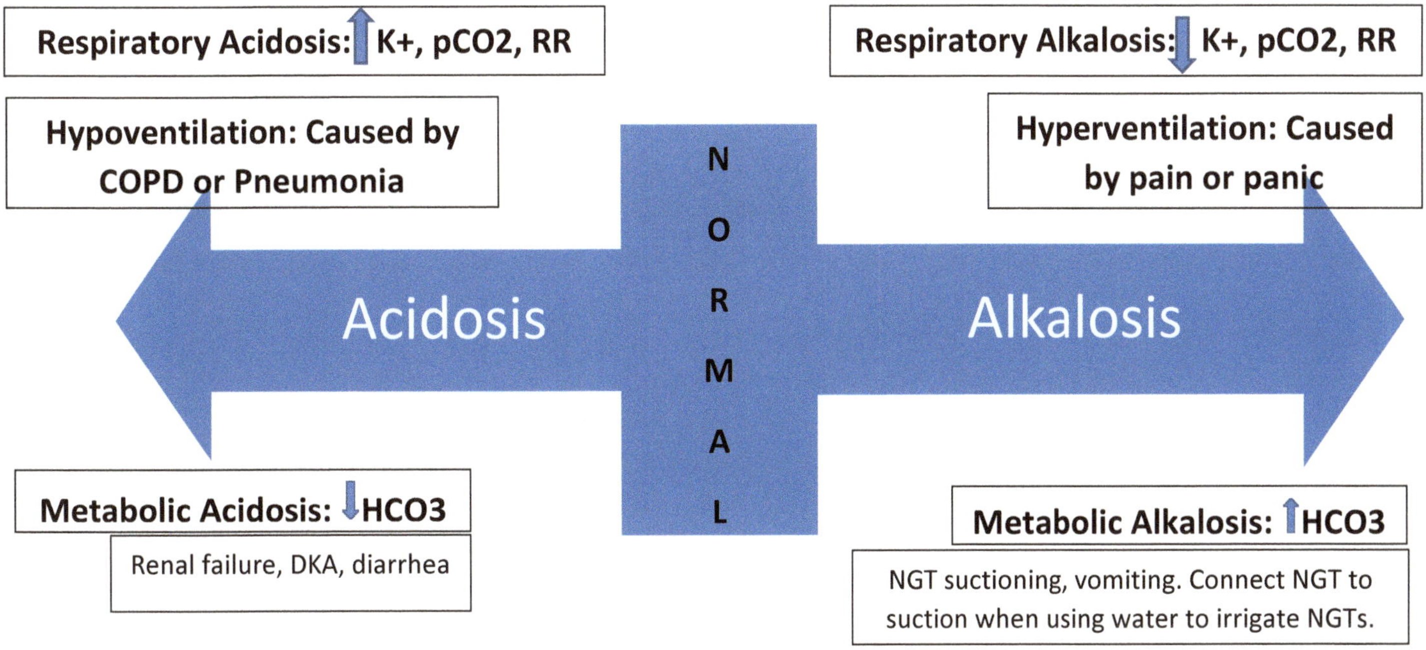

ACRONYM

Respiratory – Opposite		Metabolic- Equal	
PaCO2 ↑ and pH ↓	RESPIRATORY ACIDOSIS	HCO3 ↓ and pH ↓	METABOLIC ACIDOSIS
PaCO2 ↓ and pH ↑	RESPIRATORY ALKALOSIS	HCO3 ↑ and pH ↑	METABOLIC ALKALOSIS

A NORMAL pH REPRESENTS COMPLETECOMPENSATION.

Tic-Tac-Toe ABGs

This method helps interpret the ABGs. Memorize the normal values.

HCO3 (Bicarbonate) represents the body's metabolic state, meaning that as the HCO3 increases, the pH also increases. Antacids, diuretics, vomiting, and hyperaldosteronism cause this.

ACIDOSIS	NORMAL	ALKALOSIS (BASE)
<7.35	pH = 7.35 – 7.45 Absolute Normal = 7.40	>7.45
<22	HCO3 = 22 – 26 mEq/L Metabolic (Kidneys)	>26
	NORMAL	
>45	PaCO2 = 45 – 35 mmHg Respiratory (Lungs)	<35
PaCO2 represents the respiratory level and is the opposite of pH and HCO3.		

Look at the following exercises. They will help you interpret ABG results and understand how to determine if the patient is experiencing Respiratory or Metabolic Acidosis and Alkalosis.

Example #1

pH = 7.20

HCO3 = 28

PaCO2 = 53

ACIDOSIS	NORMAL	ALKALOSIS (BASE)
pH		HCO3
PaCO2		

PaCO2 is not normal. The patient has a <u>RESPIRATORY</u> issue.

HCO3 is not normal. The body is trying to correct itself. This means that it is <u>PARTIALLY COMPENSATED.</u>

Result: RESPIRATORY ACIDOSIS-PARTIALLY COMPENSATED

<u>Example #2</u>

pH = 7. 23

HCO3 = 24

PaCO2 = 58

ACIDOSIS	NORMAL	ALKALOSIS (BASE)
pH	HCO3	
PaCO2		

Result: RESPIRATORY ACIDOSIS-Uncompensated

<u>Example #3</u>

pH = 7.46

HCO3 = 21

PaCO2 = 30

ACIDOSIS	NORMAL	ALKALOSIS (BASE)
HCO_3		pH
		CO_2

Result: RESPIRATORY ALKALOSIS – PARTIALLY COMPENSATED

<u>Example #4</u>

pH = 7.25

HCO_3 = 18

CO_2 = 30

ACIDOSIS	NORMAL	ALKALOSIS (BASE)
		pH
	CO_2	HCO_3

Result: METABOLIC ALKALOSIS - Uncompensated

REMEMBER THAT METABOLIC REFERS TO THE KIDNEYS, AND RESPIRATORY REFERS TO THE LUNGS.

VENTILATORS

Indication for Use

When the patient presents the following signs indicating the respiratory system is compromised, the physician will order the patient to be on a ventilator:

$PaO_2<50$mmHg with $FiO_2>0.60$	$PaO_2>50$mmHg with pH<7.25	Decreased Vital Capacity	Respiratory Rate>35/min

The physician orders the setting of ventilators. The nurse monitors ABGs to determine if changes are needed. Respiratory therapists usually manage different types of ventilators.

Positive Pressure Ventilation

Positive Pressure ventilators inflate the lungs by exerting positive pressure on the airway, forcing the alveoli to expand during inspiration, followed by passive expiration. Intubation is usually necessary and can be used at home. It is used for primary lung disease.

Non-Invasive Positive Pressure Ventilation

Non-Invasive Positive Pressure Ventilation is given via face masks that cover the nose and mouth, nasal masks, and other devices. No intubation is necessary. Ventilation can be delivered by volume, pressure control, continuous positive airway device, or bilevel positive airway pressure (bi-PAP) ventilator. Pressure-controlled ventilation is the most comfortable ventilation support as it eases the work of breathing and enhances gas exchange. The Bi-PAP allows independent control of inspiratory and expiratory pressures while providing pressure-support ventilation. This device is used for ventilatory assistance at night for patients with sleep apnea or severe COPD.

Negative Pressure

This type of ventilation inflates the lungs by exerting negative pressure on the external chest, which decreases the intrathoracic pressure during inspiration, allowing air to flow into the lungs and fill its volume, similar to spontaneous ventilation. They do not require intubation and can be used at home. It is used for chronic respiratory failure related to neuromuscular conditions like Myasthenia Gravis, Polio, ALS (*amyotrophic lateral sclerosis*), or Muscular Dystrophy.

Managing Ventilator Problems

ALWAYS check the patient first when alarms sound	
Ventilator Problems	Cause
Increase in peak airway pressure. High airway pressure alarm	Coughing, plugged airway tube, patient *bucking* (something that seems oppressive or inevitable), decreasing lung compliance, tubing kinked, increased condensation in tubing, *atelectasis* (complete or partial collapse of the entire lung or lobe of the lung), bronchospasm, pneumothorax.
Low airway pressure alarm	Leaks or tubing disconnected.

Patient Problems	Cause
Cardiovascular	Decreased venous return related to positive pressure to lungs
Pneumothorax	High mean airway pressures cause alveolar collapse.
Pulmonary Infection	Frequent breaks in the ventilator circuit, decreased mobility, impaired cough, and standard defense mechanisms bypassed.

RESPIRATORY BREATH SOUNDS

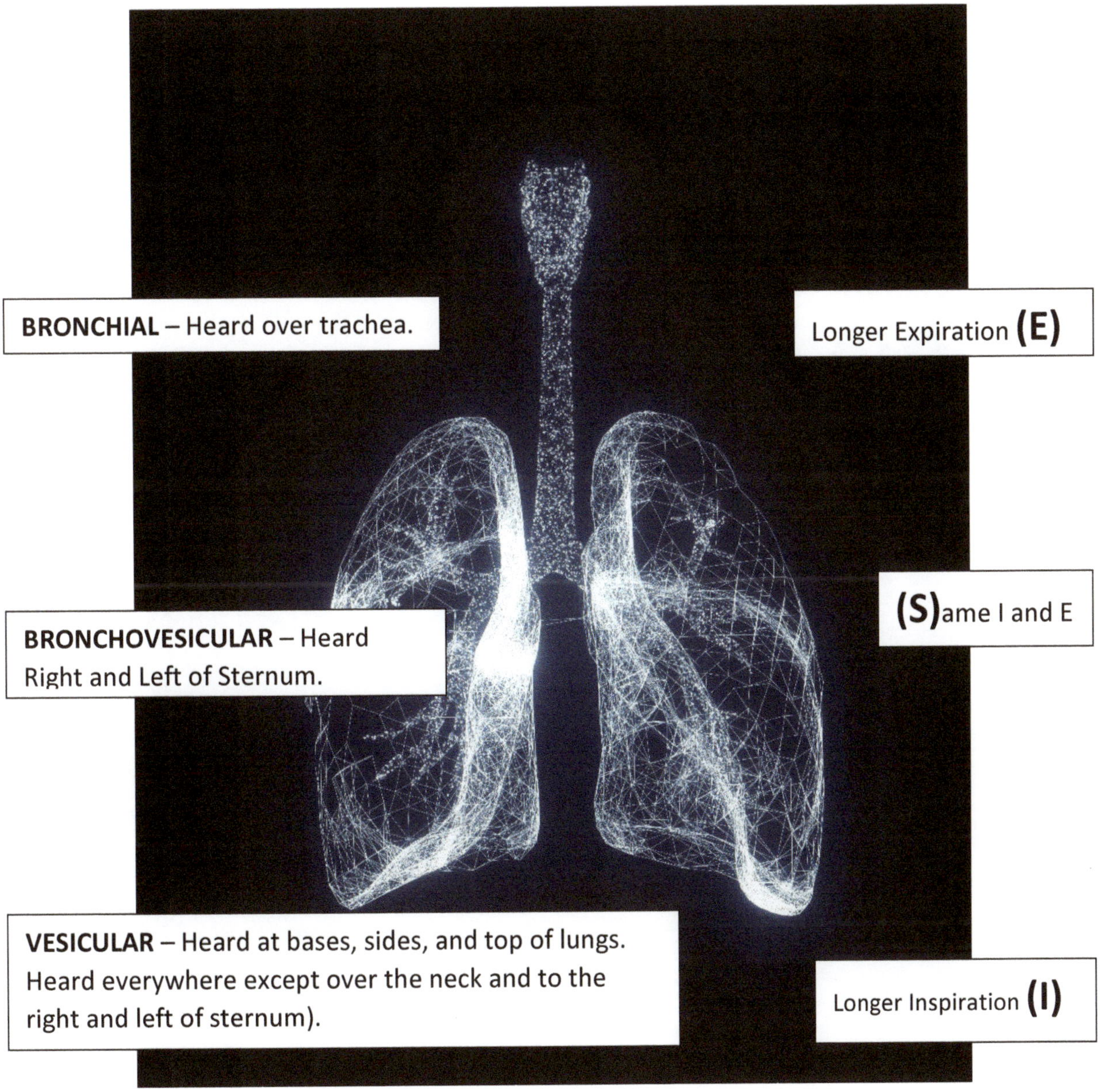

CHAPTER 5

THE ENDOCRINE SYSTEM

The endocrine system plays a crucial role in regulating the functions of various organs by secreting hormones directly into the bloodstream from its glands. These hormones are designed to reach and influence specific tissues, impacting the activity of different endocrine glands and organs throughout the body.

CONDITIONS OF THE ENDOCRINE SYSTEM

Pituitary Gland

The pituitary gland divides into two sections: anterior and posterior. The anterior part is the master gland in the body, producing the most organ-stimulating hormones.

Pituitary Hormones-Anterior	Pituitary Hormones-Posterior
TSH – Tells the thyroid to make thyroxine	ADH – *Antidiuretic Hormone*. Tells the kidney to hold onto water
ACTH – Adrenal Cortico-Trophic Hormone 1. Glucocoticosteroids (Sugar) 2. Mineralcorticosteroids (Salt) 3. Sex Hormones (Androgen and Estrogen)	Oxytocin
GH - Growth Hormones	
MSH – Melanocyte Stimulating Hormone (Skin color)	
FSH – Follicle Stimulating Hormone	
ICSH – Interstitial Cell Stimulating Hormone	
LH – Luteinizing Hormone	

DISORDERS OF THE PITUITARY

Hypopituitarism

This condition is diagnosed when a short supply of one or more hormones is identified, altering or affecting the body's normal functioning, for example, growth, reproduction, or reproduction. Causes include *atrophy* of the pituitary gland (underdeveloped) and a pituitary or brain lesion or tumor. Signs and symptoms are *hemianopia* (visual field blindness on the same side of each eye), H/A (headaches), irregular menses, *Cretinism* (if a kid, short stature, growth retardation. No effect in adults).

Possible tests that the physician will order are a skull x-ray, CT of the brain, and plasma hormone levels (T3, T4, cortisol, reproduction hormones, glucose, and sodium. Another test is the cortisol urine test. In the past, a test was ordered for the 17 hydroxy corticosteroid (17 OHCs) levels in urine. The physician used to order this test to identify if the body was producing too much cortisol (steroid) and to diagnose *Cushing syndrome*. Cushing syndrome occurs when cortisol levels in the body are constantly high.

To correct these issues, the surgeon will remove the tumor affecting the pituitary or the entire pituitary gland *(hypophysectomy)*. The patient will require hormone replacement for life. Before surgery, the physician will irradiate the tumor to shrink it.

Hyperpituitarism

A benign adenoma causes hyperpituitarism. Adenomas are not cancer but cells that develop in the epithelial tissue ("a thin layer of tissue that covers structures within the body"). Adenomas secrete tumors, causing the overproduction of pituitary hormones and resulting in hyperactive functioning of those glands. Signs and symptoms are *acromegaly* (large lips, hands, and feet in adults) and *gigantism* (tall-statured children). Other signs are *gynecomastia* (development of breasts) and *hirsutism* (development of facial hair). The diagnostic tests and treatments used for this condition are the same as those used for hypopituitarism and are described in the previous section.

Hormone Deficiency	Overproduction of Hormones
Hypothyroidism	Hyperthyroidism (*Grave's Disease)*
Diabetes Insipidus	SIADH
Fertility Problems	Fertility Problems
Cretinism (children)	Gigantism (children), Acromegaly (adults)
Addison's	Cushing's
Hypoaldosteronism (Dehydration)	Hyperaldosteronism (Volume Excess)

	HYPOPITUITARISM	HYPERPITUITARISM
Diagnostic Tests	Skull X-Ray Brain CT Hormone Levels in Plasma 24hr Urine	Same
Manifestation	Short Stature Headaches Hemianopia	Acromegaly Gigantism Hirsutism Gynecomastia
Treatment	Hypophysectomy Radiation if tumor Hormone Replacement for life	Same

HORMONE REPLACEMENT THERAPY		
Thyroxine Replacement	Synthroid, Levothyroxine	Give it before breakfast. Hold medication if BP>100
ADH	Vasopressin	
Reproductive Hormones		Replace if childbearing desire.
Growth Hormone		Replace in kids only.
Sugar Hormones	Glucocorticosteroids - Prednisone	
Salt Hormones	Mineralcorticosteroids - Florinef	

ADRENAL MEDULLA DISORDER - Hyperfunctioning

In this condition, the lower adrenal gland secretes catecholamines: Epinephrine, Norepinephrine, and Dopamine. Epinephrine (Adrenaline) and Norepinephrine (Noradrenaline) cause vasoconstriction to increase the BP.

Pheochromocytoma

Pheochromocytoma is a tumor of the adrenal medulla that causes hypersecretion of *catecholamines*. Catecholamines are neurotransmitter hormones the brain, nerve tissues, and adrenal glands produce. These hormones are epinephrine, norepinephrine, and dopamine.

Dopamine regulates movement, emotions, and memory.

Epinephrine is responsible for the fight-or-flight response to stress, increasing blood flow to muscles, the heart, and the lungs.

Norepinephrine also helps the body respond to stress, increasing heart rate and blood pressure. It is also involved in mood regulation and the ability to concentrate.

Pheochromocytoma Signs and Symptoms	
Tachycardia	Related to epinephrine (adrenaline) and norepinephrine
Hypertension	Related to epinephrine and norepinephrine
Severe headache	Related to vasoconstriction
Diaphoresis	Related to dopamine
Mydriasis	Related to epinephrine
Cold extremities	Related to epinephrine and norepinephrine

To solve these issues, the physician will order an *adrenalectomy* (removal of the adrenal gland from the top of the kidney. If only one adrenal gland is removed (*unilateral*), the patient will require hormone replacement for six months. If both adrenal glands are removed *(bilateral*), the patient will require hormone replacement for life.

Nursing Care

Nursing care includes monitoring BP and I/O and hormone replacement if necessary (glucocorticosteroids, mineral corticosteroids, and sex hormones). Patient education provides information regarding the risk of infection related to hormones and avoiding live vaccines. Patients with this condition need to make changes, including a low-calorie diet. In addition, the patient should be educated regarding the importance of taking medications in the morning with food.

Hypoaldosteronism

This condition is characterized by low aldosterone production (levels) or decreased release in the system and is a rare cause of hypertension. It can be caused by renal insufficiency, the removal of aldosterone-secreting adenomas, family history, or long-lasting administration of heparin.

Hyperaldosteronism (Conn's Syndrome)

Aldosterone is a hormone secreted by the adrenal glands that controls sodium and potassium levels in the system and regulates blood pressure. Signs and symptoms include frequent urination caused by low potassium, muscle cramps, and palpitations. Other symptoms include headache, anxiety, depression, memory loss, fatigue, and excessive thirst.

DISORDERS OF THE ADRENAL CORTEX

Addison's Disease (Hypo-functioning; Hypocortisolism; Primary Adrenal Insufficiency)

This disease is a condition in which the adrenal glands do not produce enough cortisol or aldosterone. Cortisol is an essential hormone that helps maintain blood pressure, respond to stress, and regulate heart function, the immune system, and sugar levels. *Aldosterone* is also a hormone that helps balance sodium and potassium and controls the amount of urine (fluids) discarded by the kidneys, affecting blood volume and blood pressure.

Secondary Adrenal Insufficiency occurs when the adrenal glands produce cortisol because the pituitary gland does not produce enough *adrenocorticotropic hormone* (ACTH). Too much cortisol in the system develops *Cushing's Syndrome.*

Addisonian Crisis

This condition is caused by strenuous activity, infection, stress, trauma, and abrupt cessation of steroids. The signs and symptoms are respiratory failure/distress. Treatment is airway patency, rest, and hormonal replacement.

Cushing's Syndrome (Hyperfunctioning; Hypercortisolism)

This condition develops when too much cortisol is *in the system for an extended time*. The cause is long-term use of steroids, a tumor, too many steroids after surgery (hypophysectomy or adrenalectomy), or overproduction of the adrenal glands. Classical signs and symptoms of a patient with Cushing's syndrome are the development of a fatty hump observed between the shoulders, a rounded face (weight gain), purple stretch marks on the skin, and bruises that develop quickly. The patient will also have high blood pressure, bone loss, and type 2 diabetes. The patient will have difficulty concentrating, sleeplessness, and difficulty controlling emotions.

Endogenous Cushing Syndrome occurs when the body makes too much cortisol. It may be caused by a pituitary adenoma that produces ACTH, an adrenal gland tumor or disease, family history, or the development of cancer in an organ that does not make ACTH.

Exogenous Cushing Syndrome – syndrome is caused by taking glucocorticoid (steroids) medicines used to treat lupus, rheumatoid arthritis, and asthma.

	CUSHING'S Fluid Volume Excess	ADDISON'S Fluid Volume Deficit
Manifestations	Buffalo hump Male pattern baldness Moon face (Round, Red, Full face) Hirsutism Deep voice Central obesity and purple striae Lower extremities edema	Weakness Fatigue Weight loss Decreased BP Nausea and vomiting Abdominal cramps Bronze skin (MSH increased)

Labs	Increased serum cortisol Elevated sodium Decreased potassium Glycosuria Increased 17 OCHs	Decreased serum cortisol Blood sugar Decreased sodium Increased potassium Oliguria and decreased OHCs
ECG	T-flat	QRS-wide and T-peak
Nursing Care	Intake and Output Fluid and sodium restriction Daily weight and girth Lasix Potassium supplement Check vision	#1-Monitor for respiratory failure Priority patient Intake and Output Fluids Rest-no stimuli Replace hormones forever
Diet	2gm Sodium Low CHO Low calories High protein High potassium	
Teaching		Avoid stress Avoid infections Avoid cold drafts
Medications		Glucocorticoids (sugar to have energy to breathe)
Risk	Osteoporosis and Renal Lithiasis (stones)	*Addisonian Crisis: Respiratory Failure*

THYROID DISORDERS

The thyroid is responsible for metabolism.

Diagnostic Tests	
Laboratory Tests	Preparation

T3, T4	None
TSH	None
Radioactive Iodine Uptake (RAIU) A thyroid function test	NPO for 8 hours. Discontinue thyroid medications. Discontinue iodine intake two weeks before the test. No iodine dye tests in the previous three months.
SCAN	NPO for 8 hours.

Hypothyroidism (*Myxedema*)

The thyroid gland does not produce enough thyroxine for normal metabolism in this condition. The name myxedema refers to the dermatologic changes that occur in patients with this condition. This condition is treated by replacing the thyroid hormone thyroxine. Patients must take their pulse before taking the medication before breakfast. If the pulse is >100, notify the physician and do not take the medication.

Go slow with activities. Patients may develop angina or myocardial infarction with sudden activities. Expect weight loss, decreased edema, and increased energy and appetite. Patients will not feel so cold, and their skin will not be dry anymore.

Myxedema Coma

This occurs with severe hypothyroidism and when patients stop taking the hormones. Signs and symptoms include hypothermia, bradycardia, and hypotension. Nurses must gradually maintain the patient's warmth, monitor arterial blood gases (ABGs), and replace thyroxine to achieve a therapeutic level and a functional thyroid. A low-calorie/low-fat diet is recommended. No sedatives, sleeping pills, or narcotics should be ingested because they will be metabolized slowly, increasing the sedative effect. Activities should be increased gradually.

Grave's Disease (Hyperthyroidism)

Grave's disease is an autoimmune disease causing an overproduction of thyroid hormone. Because the thyroid hormones affect many body systems, their signs and symptoms can be wide-ranging, extending to many areas. Signs and symptoms include anxiety, irritability, fine tremors of the hands or fingers, heat sensitivity, an increase in perspiration or warm, moist skin, unintended weight loss, *goiter* (enlargement of the thyroid gland), change in menstrual cycles, erectile dysfunction or reduced libido, frequent bowel movements, fatigue, sleep disturbance, and *palpitations (*rapid or irregular heartbeat).

There are two signs related explicitly to Grave's disease: *Grave's ophthalmopathy* (bulging eyes) and *Grave's dermopathy* (thick, red skin, usually on the shins or tops of the feet). Ophthalmopathy occurs from the accumulation of carbohydrates in the muscles and tissues behind the eyes. The cause is unknown.

Anti-thyroid medications are prescribed to stop the thyroid from producing thyroxine. Radioactive iodine (RAI) is used with this condition and with certain types of thyroid cancer. It can also destroy the thyroid. Lugol's solution is a medication used preoperatively to decrease *vascularity* (blood supply) to the thyroid to decrease the risk of ~~hemorrhage~~ bleeding during surgery to remove the thyroid gland. *A saturated solution of potassium iodide (SSKI) is an oral solution diluted in milk or juice to shrink the thyroid and decrease* thyroxine production. Complete or sub-total surgical removal of the thyroid is another option.

Thyroidectomy

Preoperative care: Propranolol (Inderal) to decrease heart rate and prevent pulmonary edema and Congestive Heart Failure (CHF), and Lugol's Solution to decrease vascularity. Offer the patient a tepid sponge bath or cooling blanket to reduce temperature and increase fluid intake to replace the fluids lost through diarrhea.

Post-operative care: Keep patient in semi-fowler's position. Assess dressing, back of the neck, and bed linens for bleeding. Keep tracheostomy set, oxygen, and suction at the bedside. Calcium will be low because the parathyroids are also removed, and Calcium Gluconate will be ordered to prevent tetany.

Nursing Care

Conduct tetany assessment by checking the Chvostek's (cheek) and Trousseau's (carpopedal spasm) signs. Chvostek's sign is performed by gently tapping an individual's cheek before the ear. Chvostek's sign will be positive if the facial muscles react by twitching, winking, or grimacing. Trousseau's sign is the involuntary contraction of the muscles in the hand and wrist (carpopedal spasm) that occurs after the compression of the upper arm. Place the blood pressure cuff on the upper arm and bring the dial to 150. Trousseau's sign will be positive if the wrist muscles contract.

Hyperthyroidism Crisis (Thyroid Storm)

The drastic increase in thyroid hormones causes a rare complication known as Grave's disease, which is life-threatening. It is more common when severe hyperthyroidism is inadequately treated or untreated, either by the thyroid producing too much thyroxine or too much medication given. Signs and symptoms include fever (hyperthermia), sweating, vomiting, diarrhea, delirium, weakness, seizures, irregular and severe heartbeat (tachycardia), *jaundice* (yellow skin and eyes), low BP, and coma. The patient will have severe diarrhea, losing potassium and water.

	THYROID METABOLISM			
Medications	HYPOTHYROIDISM (MYXEDEMA)	Heart Rate (60-100)	HYPERTHYROIDISM (GRAVE'S SYNDROME)	Medications
Synthroid	Increase menses. Tired, sleepy, like half-dead Difficulty in opening eyes Very cold Flaky skin – peeling Needs stimulation.	Respirations (14-20) Temperature (97.6-99.6) Activity (Rest and Activities) Peristalsis (BM q2-3 days)	Amenorrhea; Fertility problems Respirations are fast and shallow Insomnia Big eyes Very hot	Antithyroid medication Propranolol (Inderal)

	No BM – Constipation Fat remains around the heart. At risk for heart disease (CHF, MI, Angina) Low calories, low salt, high protein, low fluids No narcotics or sedatives Weight gain	Menses (q25-32 days) Weight	No stimulation Severe diarrhea Eats constantly. Weight loss	RAI (Radioactive Iodine) Surgery (Glucose Solution)

ENDOCRINE DISORDERS OF THE PANCREAS

Diabetes Mellitus (Sugar Diabetes)

Normal blood sugar (BS) is <100mg/dL. This condition is diagnosed with a Fasting Blood Sugar (FBS) that is >126mg/dL on two separate occasions. Sugar levels in the blood should not go >175 because it will put the patient at risk for cardiac diseases.

Diabetes Type I

The pancreas does not produce enough insulin to transport glucose into the cell. This condition is diagnosed during childhood. The glucose stays in the bloodstream, causing hyperglycemia. Blood glucose will be > 100. Signs and symptoms are polyuria, polyphagia (hunger), polydipsia (thirst), gradual weight loss over months, and mood changes (irritability). The patient will be prescribed insulin replacement. Patients will receive education on diet, exercise, and life changes.

TYPES OF INSULIN	*PEAK	DURATION
**Rapid-acting (R Insulins) Humulin R	It starts working within 15 min after being given. 2-4 hours	4-6 hours
Humalog; Lispro	1 hour	3 hours
Intermediate-acting (N Insulins) NPH	6-8 hours	12-20 hours

Long-acting Lantus	No peak. Steady state of glycemic control. It should be given at the same time every day, usually in the evening.	24-30 hours

*Patients can develop hypoglycemia during the peak time when the medication is working the most. Sugar should be checked at those times.

**Only R insulins can be given IV.

Diabetic Teaching

Insulin administration: NEVER change brands of insulin. Follow instructions on self-blood glucose monitoring daily, AC/HS, and as needed. Notify the physician of any changes or injuries. Skin and foot care are essential for diabetic patients. Use a nail file to smoothen the sharp corners of nails—no barefoot or colored socks. Eat small, frequent meals and snacks. It is usually recommended to have three meals and 3-4 snacks in between. Eat a carbohydrate snack before physical exercise or activity.

Signs and symptoms of *hypoglycemia* – pale, cold, clammy, crabby, shaky, weak, and headache.

Signs and symptoms of *hyperglycemia* – poly(s) – Polyuria, polydipsia, polyphagia

Diabetic Ketoacidosis (DKA)

In diabetic ketoacidosis, the pancreas does not produce enough insulin to reduce blood sugar. Glucose is high, >250mg/dL, putting the patient on *metabolic acidosis*. Signs and symptoms of DKA are polyuria, polydipsia, warm, dry, and flushed skin, nausea, vomiting, Kussmaul respirations (like blowing), and pre-coma. The physician will order an IV infusion of Regular Insulin in 0.9% NS. The blood glucose will be monitored every hour.

Diabetes Type II

This type is usually diagnosed at 35 years of age. This type is diagnosed in children. Diabetes Type II is an insulin utilization defect (lazy insulin). The pancreas produces insulin, but the insulin is not utilized to move glucose out of the bloodstream. Signs and symptoms are (polys) polyuria, polydipsia, polyphagia, obesity (patient is lazy = lazy insulin), retinopathy, neuropathy, nephropathy ("opathies"), and diabetic ulcers.

Treatment includes a calorie-restricted diet and exercise to burn off the sugar. The use of oral hypoglycemics increases the effectiveness of insulin in pushing the glucose out of the blood and into the cell. Insulin is needed if the patient is non-adherent. Oral hypoglycemics are Diabinese, Diabeta, Orinase, Tolinase, Glucotrol, Glucophage, and Avandia. Glyburide and Metformin are fast-acting medications and should be taken with meals. Teaching is the same as for Type I, except for insulin administration.

Glycosylated Hemoglobin (HGBA1c)

This blood test reveals blood glucose levels over the past three months. It shows compliance with medication, and whether the blood sugar has been stable. The ideal value is <7%

Hyperglycemic Hyperosmolar Non-Ketonic Coma

This type shows very elevated blood sugar, >300 mg/dL. This condition is usually caused by diet noncompliance. Patients with this condition tolerate high blood glucose levels better than a Type I patient. Signs and symptoms are polyuria and polydipsia. The treatment is the same as with Diabetic Ketoacidosis. The patient will receive an IV infusion of regular insulin in 0.9% NS, and the blood glucose level will be monitored every hour.

HYPOGLYCEMIA

In this condition is also known as insulin reaction and occurs when the blood glucose is <70 mg/dL. The patient will experience pallor, diaphoresis (sweating, clammy skin), cool skin, irritability (crabby), tremors and shakiness, weakness, and headache. The blood sugar must be assessed. *If the patient is alert, offer orange juice, glucose tablets, cake frosting, or hard candy. Check blood sugar 15 minutes after giving sugar. If the BG is still <70 mg/dL, repeat. Give carbohydrate snacks such as milk, cheese, crackers, or a meal tray within 30 to 60 minutes.

When the patient is stable, notify the physician about the hypoglycemic event and the treatment given. DO NOT GIVE THE NEXT DOSE OF INSULIN/ORAL HYPOGLYCEMICS UNTIL COMMUNICATING WITH THE PHYSICIAN.

*If the patient is not alert or unable to take PO, check for an order for a Dextrose 50mg ampule to give IV push. Family and significant others may be taught to administer the patient glucagon 1mg SQ or IM.

ADRENAL GLANDS

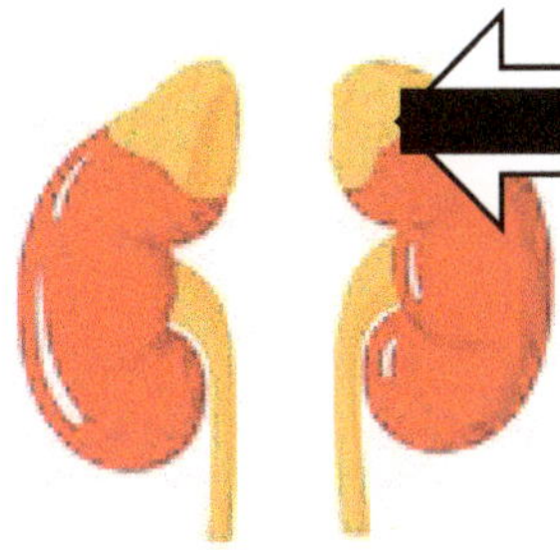

[redacted]

Located on top of each kidney.

The adrenal glands are responsible for the production and release of the following hormones: cortisol, aldosterone, DHEA and androgenic steroids, adrenaline, and noradrenaline. They are divided between catecholamines and steroids hormones.

ADDISON DISEASE

Does not have enough sugar hormone and is at risk for respiratory arrest.

CORTEX

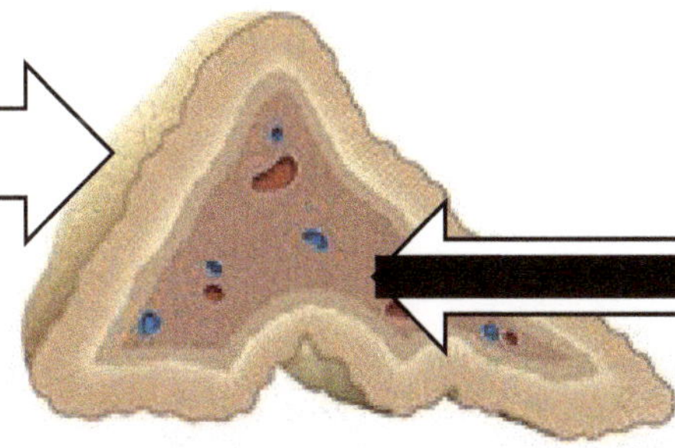

[redacted]

GLUCOCORTICOIDS (Needed to breath)

- ✓ Cortisol

MINERALCORTICOIDS

- ✓ Aldosterone

SEX STEROIDS

- ✓ Testosterone
- ✓ Endogens
- ✓ Androgens

CUSHING'S DISEASE

Patient has too much Aldosterone.

EPINEPHRINE

NOREPINEPHRINE

DOPAMINE

CHAPTER 6

THE URINARY SYSTEM

The urinary system, consisting of the kidneys, ureters, bladder, and urethra, filters the bloodstream vitally. It eliminates waste and surplus water, which is then removed from the body as urine. Moreover, this system regulates the body's internal environment, preserving homeostasis.

THE URINARY SYSTEM

The urinary system eliminates waste products cells create and maintains the body's water balance. These processes help maintain homeostasis, which is the condition in which all body systems work at their best. It comprises two kidneys, two ureters, one bladder, a single urethra, and a meatus.

Normal Changes in Aging

1. The ability to filter blood decreases.
2. The bladder muscle tone weakens.
3. The bladder holds less urine.
4. The bladder is unable to empty.

DIAGNOSTIC TESTS

LABS

Blood Urea Nitrogen (BUN) – This blood test determines the amount of urea nitrogen in the blood. Urea Nitrogen is a waste product that results when the body breaks down protein and filters it through the kidneys.

Creatinine is a waste product made when muscle tissue breaks down when the person uses the muscles and exercises. A high creatinine level in blood and urine indicates that the kidneys are malfunctioning.

Uric Acid is a chemical created when the body breaks down *purines*. Purines are found in seafood like anchovies and mackerel, alcohol, organ meats like liver, and sweetened beverages. A high level of uric acid indicates poor kidney functioning, causing some conditions such as gout and arthritis and increased risk for diabetes.

Glomerular Filtration Test (GFR) is a blood test that indicates if the kidneys are damaged if found at a high level in the blood.

X-Rays

Intravenous Pyelogram (IVP)

This test is done to diagnose obstruction. Before the test, the nurse assessed for iodine allergy (shellfish). The patient must complete a bowel preparation. After the test, the patient must be encouraged to increase fluid intake.

Kidneys, Ureters, and Bladder (KUB)

This test is an X-ray study that visualizes the urinary tract system to identify renal disorders or localize obstructions. If the test uses contrast, it is usually an iodine-based contrast. The nurse must assess any allergies the patient may have. Preparation includes fasting and bowel preparation.

Cystoscopy

This procedure allows the physician to examine and visualize the bladder, which helps diagnose BPH (*benign prostate hyperplasia*). The test is performed by inserting a cystoscope through the urethra. This thin tube with a camera helps visualize the bladder and the urethra.

Urinary Tract Infection (UTI)

Contributing factors to the development of urinary tract infections are a history of frequent infections, BPH (benign prostate hyperplasia), the bladder not emptying, changes in voiding habits, immunosuppressive therapy such as chemotherapy, unprotected sexual intercourse, use of foley catheters, and, for females, a short urethra. Signs and symptoms include fever, tachycardia, flank pain, suprapubic pain, enlargement of inguinal lymph nodes, and confusion in the elderly.

Diagnostic procedures include ultrasound, CT scans, and IV pyelogram. Signs and symptoms are treated in addition to antibiotics, increased fluids, *antipyretics* (fever reducers), and analgesics. It is essential to identify obstructions in the urinary system that prevent the patient from voiding, identify the microorganisms causing the infection, and identify any additional systemic disease.

FOODS CONTRAINDICATED FOR RENAL PATIENTS		
Baked potato Eggs	Concentrated orange juice Salt substitutes	Bananas, Apricots, Figs, Dates, Peaches (cooked or dry), Melons, Raisins, Avocados
Beans: refried, soy, kidney beans, lima beans	Coffee, Tea, Chocolate, Milk	Pumpkin
Peas, Beets, Black-eyed peas	Tomato products: paste, soup, ketchup	Nuts and seeds.

Urine Components

Components	Normal Values	Symptoms When Values Are Off
Hydrogen (H+)	1.51 g/l	Metabolic Acidosis
Ammonia (NH3)	< 30 micromol/L	Confusion if elevated.
Creatinine	(m) 0.74 to 1.35 mg/dL (w) 0,59 to 1.04 mg/dL	
Phosphorus (P)	2.5 to 4.5	P high and Ca low = *tetany,* paresthesia, and seizures.
Potassium (K+)	0.750 g/L	K+ low = *Bradycardia*
Sodium (Na)	1.17 g/L	Dehydration or fluid overload
Water (H2O)	95%	
Calcium (Ca)	8 to 10.4	
Magnesium (Mg)	1.3 to 1.5	
Urine Osmolarity	50 and 1200 mOsmol/kg	
Specific Gravity	1.002 to 1.037	

Urine pH	7.35 – 7.45	Low pH = Acidosis High pH = Alkalosis
Urea	9.3 g/dL 9 to 23 g/L	
Chloride	1.87 g/L	

Metabolic Acidosis

Some kidney conditions will create metabolic acidosis when the body produces too much acid or the kidneys are not functioning correctly and are not removing enough acid. Metabolic Acidosis is an emergency. The patient will develop *tachycardia, confusion, and fatigue*. It means that the bicarbonate level in the system is low. This condition may be caused by diabetes-related acidosis (*diabetes ketoacidosis*) when the glucose level is critically elevated. *Hyperchloremic acidosis* occurs when the body loses too much bicarbonate through diarrhea or laxatives. *Lactic acidosis* is when the patient has too much lactic acid in the system. When the system does not have enough oxygen, the muscles and the red blood cells form lactic acid.

Metabolic Alkalosis

Metabolic alkalosis is characterized by an elevated level of bicarbonate in the system. Patients who experience increased episodes of vomiting or a reduced level of acids in the system will develop metabolic alkalosis. A high intake of antacids, laxatives, baking soda, and steroids will put the patient at risk of developing metabolic alkalosis. A patient with metabolic alkalosis will experience muscle twitching, muscle cramps, and muscle spasms. Other signs and symptoms include fatigue, confusion, tremors, tingling and numbness, abnormal heart rhythm (arrhythmias), seizures, and coma. Treatment includes administration of IV saline infusion, potassium replacement, magnesium replacement, chloride infusion, and hydrochloric acid infusion. The physician may order diuretics.

FLUID IMBALANCES

Fluid imbalances occur because of dehydration (fluid deficit) or overhydration (fluid excess).

Dehydration

The HCT and the *urine-specific gravity* will be elevated. The urine-specific gravity measures the urine concentration, how the kidneys balance the water/fluids in the body, and how well they eliminate toxins and other waste. It measures the electrolytes in the urine. The normal specific gravity is 1.010 to 1.025. Another test is the *urine osmolality*. This test measures the amount of chloride, glucose, sodium, potassium, and urea in the urine. Treatment is the replacement of fluids. Depending on the severity of the condition, fluids might be ordered to be given through the vein.

Overhydration

Signs and symptoms of overhydration are *pitting sacral edema* and *crackles.* Pitting edema is fluid accumulation, more frequently found in the legs, ankles, and feet. It can also occur ~~in~~ the lower back when the sacrum and vertebrae get swollen due to fluid accumulation or from being in bed for a long time. An indentation is formed when pressure is applied over the swollen area.

Crackles are the sounds heard when the lungs are auscultated. This is a sign of fluid overload affecting the lungs. Patients are administered diuretics to eliminate or decrease the amount of fluid in the system. If the kidneys are not functioning correctly, patients may be put on *dialysis*.

Fine Crackles Sounds (EMTprep.com) - https://youtu.be/Vle350pTl8Q

Coarse Crackles Sounds (EMTprep.com) - https://youtu.be/z2Ra9UxndI0

ELECTROLYTES IMBALANCES

Electrolytes are substances with positive or negative electrical charges. The adult body is about 60% water. The electrolyte charges are activated when the electrolytes are dissolved in water. They act like batteries by triggering and regulating chemical reactions. Electrolytes are obtained through food and fluid intake and help maintain chemical balance in the body.

Potassium Imbalance

Potassium (K+) is necessary for all neuromuscular functions in the body, especially heart function. 80% of K+ is excreted by urine, and 20% of K+ lives in the GI system.

Potassium - Normal value in blood – 3.5 to 5.0 mEq/L

	HYPOKALEMIA <3.2mEq/L	HYPERKALEMIA >5.5 mEq/L
Causes	Diuretics, Burns, Diarrhea, Vomiting, Cushing's Syndrome, Steroids, NGT Suctioning	Renal Failure, Potassium Supplements, NSAIDS, Addison's Syndrome
Signs and Symptoms	Muscle weakness, Confusion, Vomiting	Same as hypokalemia
ECG	Tachycardia, PVCs, Flat T wave *Low K+ = Low T wave and High Pulse*	Bradycardia, PVCs, wide QRS, peaked T-wave *High K+ = High T wave and Low Pulse*
Treatment	Replace potassium.	Remove potassium
Other Considerations	A diet rich in potassium foods. Glucose + Regular Insulin (pushes the K+ back into the blood). Administer Calcium Glutamate IV pushes to protect the heart. At risk for falls.	Administer *Kayexalate* (pushes K+ out of the body). If Kayexalate enema is given a cleansing enema, it is necessary. At risk of falling.

Sodium Imbalance

Sodium is essential to maintain body fluid balance and help cells absorb nutrients.

Sodium - Normal value in blood – 136 to 145 mmol/L

	HYPONATREMIA < 135 mmol/L	HYPERNATREMIA >145 mmol/L
Causes	Vomiting, Increased perspiration, Renal Failure, dilution, SIADH	Diarrhea, IV 0.9 NS (Normal Saline), Decreased water intake
Signs and Symptoms	Cool and moist skin, low BP, low urine output, headaches, nausea, vomiting, weight loss, Confusion	THIRST, dry and sticky mucous membranes, fever, *oliguria*, edema, confusion, fever
ECG	No impact was observed on the ECG.	

Treatment	Administer IV fluids: 0.9 NS, Lactated Ringer (LR), or D5/0.9 NS; use NS for irrigation; include broth/bouillon in the diet.	Dilute sodium (Na+) with D5/W IV. Increase water intake
Other Considerations	N/A	N/A

Calcium Imbalances

Calcium is essential to building bones and teeth, controlling muscle movement, transmitting nerve signals, and managing the heart rhythm. Normal calcium levels in the blood are between 8.6 and 10.3 mg/dL. Signs and symptoms of calcium imbalances are:

Hypocalcemia – <8.2 mg/dL. The leading causes are abnormal levels of vitamin D and low levels of *parathyroid hormone* (referred to as the *"calcium thermostat of the body."* Hypocalcemia can cause arrhythmias, seizures, tetany, heart block, hypotension, and *laryngospasm*. Laryngospasm is the sudden involuntary constriction blocking the vocal cords.

Hypercalcemia- > 10.5 mg/dL - The leading causes of hypercalcemia are overactive parathyroid glands, high levels of vitamin D and calcium supplements in the blood, and cancer. A patient with *Addison's Disease* (adrenal insufficiency) can develop hypercalcemia. A patient's kidneys with a high calcium level in the blood must work harder to eliminate the toxins in the system. The patients will experience constipation more frequently. Because the extra calcium in the blood comes from the bones, the patients will experience bone pain and weakness. As a result, the patients will complain of palpitations and fainting caused by arrhythmias. An excess of calcium will also impact the brain. Patients will also experience confusion, lethargy, and fatigue, including depression. Treatment will be related to the cause.

Bicarbonate Imbalance

Bicarbonate is recycled carbon dioxide. The body uses bicarbonate to maintain normal blood pH levels.

Acidosis—A bicarbonate level below 22 indicates the blood is more acidic, and it is called acidosis. Signs and symptoms of acidosis are confusion, fatigue, nausea, and vomiting. The patient's respirations will be faster and deeper.

Alkalosis - A bicarbonate level above 26 indicates the blood is more alkaline, and it is called *alkalosis*. Signs and symptoms of alkalosis are confusion, arrhythmias, and muscle twitching.

Chloride Imbalances

Chloride is essential to maintain the pH level in the blood balance.

Hypochloremia—Too much chloride in the body causes the blood to be alkaline, which relates to hyponatremia. Signs and symptoms include confusion, arrhythmias, and muscle twitching.

Hyperchloremia causes the blood to be more acidic. The signs and symptoms depend on the cause because hyperchloremia is usually associated with hypokalemia or hyperkalemia. If associated with hypokalemia, the patient will present diarrhea and urinary tract issues. If associated with hyperkalemia, the patient will have severe kidney issues or kidney failure.

URINARY TRACT SURGERIES

Nephrostomy Tube

This procedure drains urine from the kidneys. Kidney stones, infections, injury, or trauma may cause this. The tube is temporary and may remain in place for days or months.

Nursing Care

After surgery, approximately 30 ml of urine should be drained in an hour. The dressing change is sterile because it is at risk for infection. The surgeon changes the tube approximately every three months.

Kidney Transplant

Patients with renal failure will eventually need a kidney transplant.

Nursing Care

Keep the patient in isolation and monitor intake and output closely. Encourage patients to drink eight ounces of water a day. The specific gravity level will be between 1.004 and 1.005. Patients will have sudden urine output but will remain in dialysis until the kidney starts to filter urine. After the transplant, the patients will be on immunosuppressing medications to prevent rejection. The risk time is from four months to four years. Signs and symptoms of rejection are *fever, pelvic pain, and decreased urine output*.

Nephrectomy

This procedure involves removing a kidney. The remaining kidney should take over the function of both kidneys. A complication of this procedure is renal failure.

UROLITHIASIS/NEPHROLITHIASIS

They are commonly known as kidney stones. Deposits of minerals and salts form and harden in the kidneys because of urine concentration. Passing kidney stones can be painful, depending on their size and irregular shape, and generally affect the urinary system. If the stones get stuck or lodged in the urinary system, an infection develops, or additional complications occur, the patients will require surgery.

Patients often require *lithotripsy*, a noninvasive procedure. The nephrologist visualizes the stone lodged in the urinary system using an ultrasound. Ultrasonic waves of energy are sent to destroy the stone into small pieces. A complication of this procedure is bleeding in the intestines and colon damage. The nephrologist should be notified immediately if bruising is noticed.

Patients frequently developing urinary tract infections (UTIs) are at risk for kidney stones. This is because urine is alkaline when a UTI develops. Kidney stones are also more prevalent during the summer because people forget to increase their water consumption and become dehydrated.

Nursing Care

Signs and symptoms are pain and vomiting. The primary intervention is providing comfort and pain management. The urine is strained to identify what kind of stone it is. Ambulation is encouraged to help move the stone. Increase fluid intake. Dairy product intake should be decreased, and fruit and veggie intake should be increased. These interventions will help reduce the development of calcium stones.

RENAL FAILURE/INJURY

Acute and Chronic

General signs and symptoms of acute renal failure/injury are decreased urine output, chest pain or pressure, jugular vein distention, fluid retention (evidenced by edema on legs, ankles, or feet), shortness of breath, confusion, nausea, seizures, or coma depending on the severity of the situation. (Refer to the following table).

Pre-Renal

When the kidneys fail to filter the urine, waste accumulates in the blood. This happens when the blood supply to the kidneys is blocked, direct damage to the kidneys through a traumatic event, or ureters are blocked, and waste cannot be excreted. Some conditions that can interfere with kidney function are *Congestive Heart Failure* (CHF), *Myocardial Infarction* (MI), and severe GI bleeding. Diabetes and hypertension (HTN) put patients at high risk for the development of renal failure.

Intra-Renal *(Most Common)*

Other reasons could include radioisotopes, dyes utilized during X-rays and other diagnostic tests, anesthetics, and frequent urinary tract infections. Radioisotopes are unstable components that emit radiation to become more stable. They are used in medicine to destroy diseased cells, like cancer cells.

Acute and Chronic renal failure can also result from receiving aminoglycoside antibiotics. These antibiotics are nephrotoxic, causing the renal tubules to become necrotic. Renal tubules are very sensitive to a decrease in blood flow. Frequent and multiple administration of these antibiotics is not recommended.

Aminoglycoside Antibiotics (suffix *"mycin")*			
Vancomycin	Tobramycin	Neomycin	Paromomycin
Gentamycin	Streptomycin	Kanamycin	*Cortisporin*

Post-Renal

Kidney stones are a post-renal cause of acute kidney failure. The urine is blocked by the stones, creating other complications, resulting in kidney failure.

Renal Failure Phases

Onset Phase – Kidney injury occurs.

Phase I – *Oliguric/Anuric phase.* In this phase, urine output is reduced to approximately < 400mlin 24 hours. Patients may develop *metabolic alkalosis.* Metabolic Alkalosis is critical. To function correctly, the blood should have an acidic/alkali balance. If this balance is interrupted, the person will become sick. *Alkalosis* means there is an elevation of *bicarbonate* level in the system.

Phase II—Diuretic Phase. In this phase, the kidneys try to heal, and approximately 10% of the kidneys try to work again and eliminate urine. However, when this happens, the kidneys can be damaged even more. It is characterized by a fluid-volume deficit (hypovolemia), and the patients should not have fluid restrictions. During this phase, it is challenging to keep the heart rate up.

Recovery Phase – Kidneys eliminate the toxins and recover functionality.

Types of AKI

TYPES OF ACUTE KIDNEY INJURY (AKI)	
TYPE	CAUSE
Pre-renal Injury It decreased renal blood flow.	1. Sepsis, trauma, bleeding, or poor cardiac output. 2. Use of nonsteroidal anti-inflammatory agents (NSAIDs) • Advil • Motrin • Aleve (Naproxen) 3. Use of cyclooxygenase (COX-2) inhibitors • Celebrex (Only one available in the US) 4. NSAIDs are called nonselective NSAIDs because they block the action of both COX 1 and 2 enzymes. • COX 1 enzyme – Produces prostaglandins that help protect the stomach and intestinal tract from digestive acids. They also help control blood clotting. • COX 2 enzyme – Produces prostaglandins involved in inflammation. 5. The prolonged use of these medications inhibits the action of COX-1 and COX-2, triggering vasoconstriction in renal arterioles and decreasing the glomerular filtration rate.
Intrinsic Injury Acute tubular necrosis.	1. Sepsis and Renal Ischemia • Renal ischemia results from a low MAP (mean arterial pressure) below 70 mm Hg. This creates poor organ perfusion and multisystem failure. 2. Nephropathy – caused by contrast agents.

	3.	Aminoglycoside Therapy – These antibiotics are poorly absorbed when given orally. Administration should be IV -They are excreted through the kidneys. If the dose is not monitored, it will damage the tubules. • Amikacin • Gentamicin • Neomycin • Streptomycin • Tobramycin
Postrenal Injury Obstructive nephropathy.	1.	Mechanical obstruction of urine flow • Kidney stones (renal calculi) • Tumors • BPH • Strictures (narrowing) • Congenital disabilities

AKI Phases

FOUR PHASES OF ACUTE KIDNEY INJURY		
PHASE	FEATURES	DURATION
Onset Phase Triggered by: Blood loss Burns Fluid loss Diabetes Insipidus	Blood flow to the kidneys is 25% of normal flow. Tissue oxygenation is also 25% of normal. Urine output is below 0.5 mL/kg/hour.	Hours - Days
Oliguric (Anuric) Phase Urine output is below 400 mL/day (it could go as low as 100 mL/day)	Increased BUN and Creatinine levels in the blood. Kidneys cannot excrete water, developing electrolyte imbalances, metabolic acidosis, and fluid overload.	8 to 14 days or longer.

Diuretic Phase It occurs when AKI is treated and corrected.	Renal tubule scarring and edema. Increased glomerular filtration (GFR) Daily urine output > 400 mL Electrolyte depletion from increased fluid intake. BUN decreases due to a better osmotic effect	7 to 14 days
Recovery Phase	Decreased edema. Normal level of fluids and electrolyte balance GFR back to 70% to 80% normal	Several months to 1 year.

Nursing Care

1. Skin—Renal patients may complain of itchy skin, gout, and breaks. Their skin may also show a bronzy tone.

2. Mental Status – Patients will be confused if the toxins levels are elevated.

3. Weight—When the kidneys are not functioning well, the patient will retain fluids. The best way to know this is by weighing the patient.

4. Vital Signs—The patients are at risk for developing pericarditis. Pericarditis is the inflammation of the pericardium, the sac that surrounds the heart and keeps it in place. High temperature is a sign that pericarditis might be developing. If the heart is auscultated, there will be a distinct sound known as *pericardial friction rub.*

Another complication is *cardiac tamponade*. Cardiac tamponade occurs when the heart's lining accumulates fluid, putting pressure on the heart. This pressure limits the amount of blood that can be pumped, as evidenced by a drop in BP. Cardiac Tamponade is fatal if it is not resolved.

Pericardial Friction Rub Sound

https://youtu.be/B2FEmI5RYHE

1. I & O – The output of a patient with kidney failure will be approximately 500ml/24 hours.
2. Diet – The diet should be low in sodium, protein, and potassium. The diet should be high in carbohydrates.
3. Medications - Remember the 3 "Ds": *Dehydration, Drugs, Diuretics*
    - Calcium supplements and vitamin D – Prevent tetany.
    - Diuretics
    - Phosphate binders – Aluminum antacids bind the phosphorus to prevent its absorption, causing *hyperphosphatemia.*
    - Stool softeners – Cause the patients to retain potassium.
    - Epogen – Given to patients on dialysis who are anemic. It acts like the hormone-producing red blood cells.

As the condition progresses, the patients will require *dialysis* or kidney transplants.

DIALYSIS

When the kidneys cannot process waste and work properly, patients are put on dialysis. In dialysis, the patients are connected to a machine three days a week for approximately three to four hours to do the kidneys' job. While in dialysis, the patients must continue to take their medications and follow a diet regime. There are two types of dialysis.

Hemodialysis

Before starting hemodialysis, the patient will undergo a surgical procedure to create access to connect the machine. Accesses are considered the "lifeline" for treatment. There are three access devices: arteriovenous (AV) grafts, AV fistulas*, or central line catheters.*

- AV graft –A tube connects the artery to the vein. It goes from the high-flow (artery) into the low-flow (vein). This is usually placed in the arm but can also be placed on the leg.
- AV fistula: An artery is connected directly to a vein to maintain the flow from high to low.
- Central Line Catheters—These are not permanent solutions. They are used until the patient receives a graft or fistula. This Y-shaped catheter can be inserted into the arm, neck, or groin. Placing it in the groin is not encouraged due to the increased infection risk. The catheter enters an artery, and the other end exits the skin to connect the dialysis machine. Catheter care is critical, and sterile techniques should be followed.

Peritoneal Dialysis (PD)

This type of dialysis uses the lining of the abdomen as a filter. A peritoneal catheter is placed into the abdomen. A cleansing fluid is drained inside the abdomen, and the filtered waste flows out afterward. This process can be done at home.

Nursing Care

The patency of the graft/fistula should be assessed frequently. This is done by checking the bruit (sound) and the thrill (feeling). Patients' BP or venipuncture should not be performed in an extremity with an AV fistula or graft.

AV Fistula Bruit - https://youtu.be/7L1bZr6aQz4

Patients should be weighed pre- and post-dialysis. Some medications, such as BP medications, should be held. Vital signs are assessed when the patient is connected to the dialysis machine. Assessment of equilibrium is also critical. Diet education is essential for these patients. Patients on peritoneal dialysis (PD) need to care for the catheter to prevent complications. Catheter care should follow the sterile technique.

KIDNEY TRANSPLANT

Patients with renal failure or *End-Stage Renal Disease* (ESRD) will eventually need a kidney transplant. A healthy kidney is removed from a living or deceased person to replace the damaged kidney of another person.

Nursing Care

Keep the patient in isolation and monitor intake and output closely. Encourage patients to drink eight ounces of water a day. The specific gravity level will be between 1.004 and 1.005. Patients will have sudden urine output but will remain in dialysis until the kidney starts to filter urine. After the transplant, the patients will be on immunosuppressing medications to prevent rejection. The risk time is from four months to four years. Signs and symptoms of rejection are *fever, pelvic pain, and decreased urine output*.

BENIGN PROSTATIC HYPERTROPHY/HYPERPLASIA (BPH)

In this condition, the prostate becomes enlarged, narrowing the urethra and preventing the patient from voiding. Signs and symptoms include hesitancy, nocturia, frequency, urgency, and dysuria. Because of urgency, the patient may complain of "drippling" or incontinence.

This is diagnosed through DRE (digital rectal examination), ultrasound, cystoscopy (urinary endoscopy), and PSA (blood test). PSA normal values are between 0 and 2.0 ng/mL. This condition is a risk factor for *prostate cancer.* It is essential to mention that prostate cancer is more aggressive in young men.

Sometimes, patients require a surgical procedure called *Transurethral Resection of the Prostate* (TURP). This procedure removes excess tissue. The risk of this procedure is bleeding. As technological advances evolve, patients have other options, such as laser surgery.

Another treatment is *Continuous Bladder Irrigation* (CBI). This procedure removes and prevents blood clots in the bladder and removes urine accumulated in it.

Some patients take *Saw Palmetto.* Saw Palmetto is an herbal supplement that should be taken with food. It is also nephrotoxic. It helps to stop nocturia.

Prostate Cancer Surgery

The treatment is *perineal prostatectomy*, which involves removing the prostate. A tube is placed through the abdomen, above the pubic bone (suprapubic), and into the bladder. The main risk is bleeding, and the patient is at risk of hemorrhaging. Within eight hours after the surgery, the patient should void.

Nursing Care

After the surgery, the nurse should assess for bleeding and *shock.* If blood flow is reduced or blocked, the patient could go into shock. Medication intake is also essential. Education should include continence, activities, and sexual function. To assist with sexual function, the patient will learn how to perform perineal exercises (Kegel Exercises). These exercises will help with sphincter control and should be started two weeks after surgery.

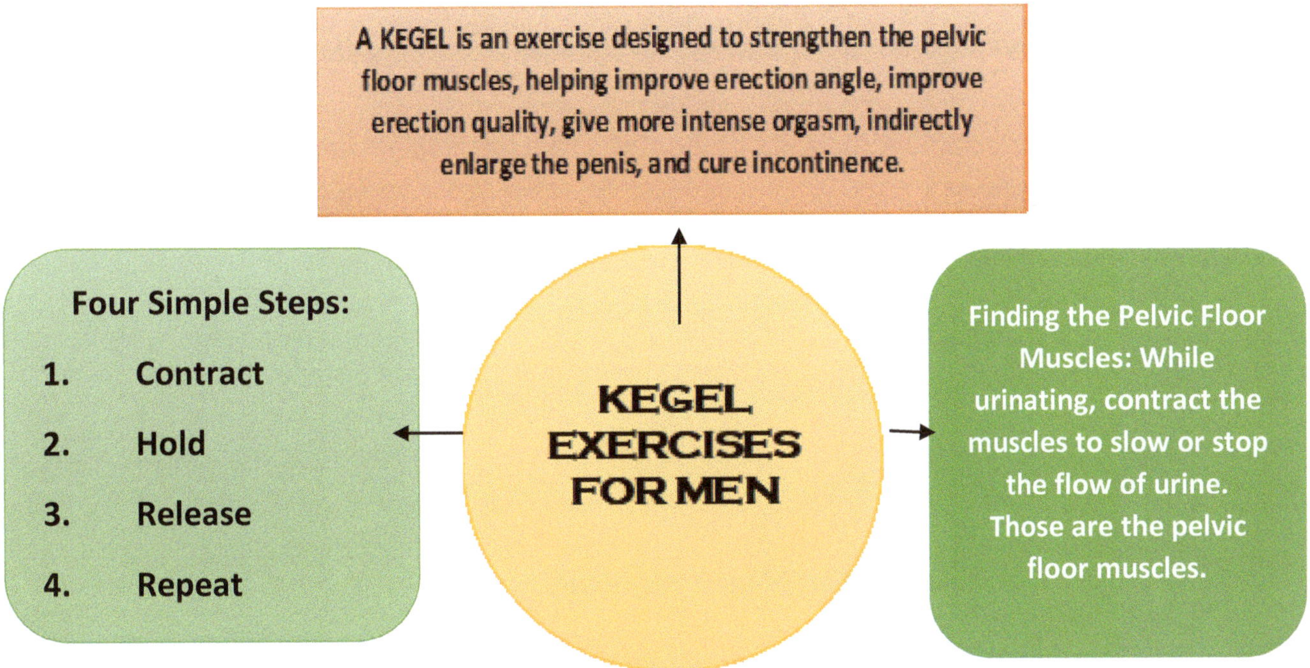

VASECTOMY

This is a permanent sterilization or birth control for men. The procedure cuts the sperm from reaching the semen.

Nursing Care

Instruct the patient to ice the area, use scrotal support, no sex for one to two weeks, light activity, contraceptive use until two ejaculate specimens test negative for sperm *motility* (movement).

BLADDER CANCER

Bladder cancer is more common in women. The first sign is painless hematuria. Risk factors include UTIs, prostate cancer, history of smoking, environmental toxins, rubber, dye or ink, tanning, and paint. The prognosis is poor if not diagnosed in the early stage.

ERECTILE DYSFUNCTION (ED)

Erectile dysfunction is also known as impotence. It is the inability to get or keep an erection long enough for intercourse. The patient will complain of reduced sexual desire. Patients can take medication; however, they need to be educated that if the erection takes longer than four hours, they should go to the emergency room. Side effects of the medications include headaches, nausea, diarrhea, and eye problems resulting in blindness.

CHAPTER 7 THE REPRODUCTIVE SYSTEM

The reproductive system is made up of organs and structures vital for reproduction. In males, it includes the testes, penis, seminal vesicles, prostate, and urethra. In females, the system is composed of the ovaries, fallopian tubes, uterus, vagina, and vulva. As males age, they may experience a decline in sperm production and an enlargement of the prostate. Females, on the other hand,

"This system comprises tissues, glands, and organs involved in producing offspring (children). In women, the reproductive system includes the ovaries, the fallopian tubes, the uterus, the cervix, and the vagina. In men, it includes the prostate, the testes, and the penis."

CONDITIONS AND DISEASES OF THE REPRODUCTIVE SYSTEM

Female

Endometriosis

Endometriosis is when tissue covering the uterus lining grows in other areas, such as the ovaries, behind the uterus, on the bowels, or the bladder. Signs and symptoms include abdominal pain, lower back pain, pain in pelvic areas, infertility, and heavy periods.

Uterine Fibroids

Uterine fibroids are common noncancerous tumors in women of childbearing age. They are made of muscle cells and other tissues that grow in and around the walls of the uterus. Signs and Symptoms include heavy and painful periods with bleeding between periods, feeling "full" in the lower abdomen, urinary frequency, painful intercourse, lower back pain, and reproductive problems, such as infertility, multiple miscarriages, or early labor.

Gynecologic Cancer

There are five primary gynecologic cancers: cervical, ovarian, uterine, vaginal, and vulvar.

Human Immunodeficiency Virus (HIV)/ Acquired Immune Deficiency Syndrome (AIDS)

The human immunodeficiency virus affects specific immune system cells (CD4 cells). Over time, the body cannot fight off infection anymore. Acquired immune deficiency syndrome is the late stage of HIV. Women are infected with HIV by having sex with an infected man or by sharing needles with an infected person.

Interstitial Cystitis (IC)

Interstitial cystitis is a chronic bladder condition characterized by inflamed or irritated bladder walls that can cause scarring and stiffening of the bladder. Interstitial cystitis can also affect men, but this condition is more prevalent in women. Signs and symptoms include abdominal or pelvic mild discomfort, urinary frequency, urinary urgency, abdominal or pelvic pressure, tenderness, intense pain in the bladder or pelvic region, and severe lower abdominal pain that intensifies as the urinary bladder fills or empties.

Polycystic Ovary Syndrome (PCOS)

Polycystic Ovary Syndrome occurs when a woman's ovaries or adrenal glands produce more male hormones than usual, causing fluid-filled sacs (cysts) to develop on the ovaries. This condition is a risk factor for diabetes and heart disease. Signs and Symptoms include infertility, pelvic pain, excess hair growth on the face, chest, stomach, thumbs, or toes, baldness or thinning hair, acne, oily skin, dandruff, or thickened dark brown or black skin patches.

Sexually Transmitted Diseases (STDs)

Sexually transmitted diseases (STDs) are bacteria, parasites, and viruses that women get from having sex with someone who has the infection. There are more than 20 types of STDs. The more common types are chlamydia, herpes, gonorrhea, HIV, HPV, syphilis, and trichomoniasis. There is no cure for STDs caused by a virus.

Sexual Violence (SV)

Sexual violence is a sexual activity where consent is not freely given. Anyone can be a victim of sexual violence, but most of the victims are women.

Intimate Partner Violence (IPV)

This is sexual violence that a current or former partner or spouse inflicts on the victim. This can occur in heterosexual or homosexual relationships. Does not require sexual intimacy.

Male

Testicular Cancer

Abnormal growth of cells develops in the testes. Testes are organs that make sperm and the hormone *testosterone*. They are inside the scrotum behind the penis. The patient will feel a lump that proliferates, usually in one testicle, prompting the patient to seek medical advice. Testicular cancer cause is unknown and can grow to other parts of the body. Testicular cancer is not common but is treatable. Signs and symptoms include a feeling of heaviness in the scrotum, dull ache in the lower belly or groin, sudden swelling in the scrotum, pain or discomfort in a testicle or the scrotum, enlargement or tenderness of the breast tissue, and back pain. A risk factor is the history of *cryptorchidism*. Cryptorchidism is having an undescended testicle. Other factors are family history, being 15 to 45 years old, and being white. Treatment is chemotherapy and surgery.

Nursing Care

Patient education on prevention is the best intervention. Explain to the patient about the importance of self-examination.

Cancer of the Penis (Penile Cancer)

Penile cancer is rare, but if discovered early on, it is treatable. Ninety-five percent of penile cancer cases are *squamous cell carcinoma*. Other cancers that could develop are *sarcoma, melanoma,* and *basal cell carcinoma*. Risk factors include a history of human papillomavirus (HPV), HIV, or AIDS; the patients are not circumcised; phimosis and *psoriasis* treatment with the drug *psoralen* and ultraviolet (UV) light.

Signs and symptoms may include changes in skin thickness or color, such as bluish-brown growths, rash or small crusty bumps on your penis, bad-smelling discharge (*smegma*), bleeding sore on the penis, and swelling at the end of the penis. Besides chemotherapy or radiation, treatment includes penectomy, laser, surgery of damaged cells, cryotherapy, and circumcision.

Phimosis (Foreskin Problems)

This is a condition that may affect children and adults who are not circumcised, where the foreskin cannot be pulled back. This condition could appear if a condition called *balanitis xerotica obliterans (BXO)* develops. *Balanitis Xerotica Obliterans* is when the skin hardens and swells with purple, white, grey, or red discoloration. It is painful and develops on the head of the penis. This condition is linked to penile cancer.

Testicular Torsion

When the testicle hangs in the scrotum, the spermatic cord in the testicle twists around, blocking the blood supply and developing testicular torsion. This is an emergency. If this condition is not addressed within six hours, the testicle could die, leading to infertility. Other signs and symptoms include a visible lump on one or both testicles, one higher than the other, scrotum discoloration (red, purple, brown, black), nausea and vomiting, and abdominal pain. Fever will appear, and the patient may be voiding more than usual.

Male Infertility

Approximately ten to fifteen percent of couples in the United States are infertile. In men, causes vary, from low sperm count and problems with the delivery of sperm to a history of cancer. Environmental factors are also considered risk factors, such as tobacco and alcohol use, obesity, and lack of exercise. Some medications can also affect fertility in men.

Erectile Dysfunction (ED)

This is the inability to keep an erection long enough for sex. Causes include heart disease and atherosclerosis, high cholesterol, low testosterone level, HTN, and diabetes. Parkinson's disease and Multiple sclerosis are common causes of ED. *Peyronie's disease* (development of scar tissue inside the penis) is often associated with ED. Surgeries that affect the spinal cord can also affect ED. In many cases, this condition can be treated with medications. Erectile dysfunction will result in psychological issues, such as anxiety, depression, and relationship problems.

Priapism

When the blood remains in the penis and is unable to be drained, the patient experiences a painful erection that occurs without stimulation and lasts hours. There are three types of priapism. This condition is a risk factor for erectile dysfunction.

Low-flow—the blood remains in the erection chambers. This is the most common type. A diagnosis of sickle cell, leukemia, Thalassemia, recreational drug use, or malaria puts the patient at risk for developing this condition. The use of some medications, such as antidepressants and antipsychotics, is also a cause of this condition.

Recurrent – A type of low-flow that goes away and comes back. It stays longer and is more painful every time.

High-Flow – This type is rare and not painful. This type develops after injury between the scrotum and the perineum (anus).

Treatment options for this condition include draining the blood from the penis, medication like NSAIDs, use of an ice pack to reduce the swelling, and surgery. Light exercise and hydration help lessen the pain. The patient should be advised not to masturbate.

VASECTOMY

This is a permanent sterilization or birth control for men. The procedure cuts the sperm from reaching the semen.

Nursing Care

Instruct the patient to ice the area, use scrotal support, no sex for one to two weeks, light activity, contraceptive use until two ejaculate specimens test negative for sperm *motility* (movement).

CHAPTER 8

THE GASTROINTESTINAL SYSTEM

The gastrointestinal system, also known as the digestive system, is a complex network of organs that work together to ingest food and liquids, break them down into nutrients for energy, growth, and repair, and then expel the unusable waste through bowel movements. This system includes the mouth, throat, esophagus, stomach, small and large intestines, rectum, and anus, along with the salivary glands, liver,

DIAGNOSTIC TESTS

Upper Gastrointestinal Series (UGI) – Barium Swallow

This test assesses the esophagus and the stomach. The patient must be NPO for at least six hours before the test. After the test, the patient will receive laxatives and fluids. Expect chalky stools within twenty-four hours.

Lower Gastrointestinal Series (LGI) – Barium enema

This test assesses the colon (large intestine). Before the test, the patient ingests a bowel preparation at approximately noon on the day. The diet must be a low residue or liquid the night before the test. The patient must be NPO for six hours before the test. This is an uncomfortable test. Reassure the patient that heshe will be able to have a BM after.

After the test, the physician will order laxatives. Increase fluid intake. Patients should have a BM within twenty-four hours after the test.

Esophagogastroduodenoscopy (EGD) - Endoscopy

This test assesses the esophagus, stomach, and duodenum. Patients must be NPO. After the test, the nurse assesses the patient for *dyspnea* (difficulty breathing), gag reflex, sore throat, and swallowing. Patients experience some hoarseness.

Sigmoidoscopy

This test assesses the lower end of the colon. The patient receives a bowel preparation before the test. After the test, the most important thing is to evaluate for bleeding.

Colonoscopy

This test assesses the colon (large intestine). The care offered before this test is the same as for LGI. Air is instilled inside the colon during the test before the scope is inserted. After the test, also assess for bleeding.

Gastric Analysis

This test consists of aspiration of gastric secretions to identify problems with the secretory potential of the stomach. It is performed without stimulation up to the stomach's maximum secretory ability with stimulation. It is ordered for patients who experience diarrhea, constipation, bloating, and other gastric symptoms.

Ultrasound of Gallbladder, Liver, Pancreas

This is not an invasive test. Before the ultrasound, patients are required to remain NPO. There is no bowel preparation, and the patient will not experience pain. The test is performed using high-frequency sound waves; the technician observes the organs to identify anomalies.

Liver Biopsy

A biopsy consists of the aspiration of a sample of liver tissue. If the patient goes through this test, the patient does not have enough clotting factor. It is essential to assess the PT/INR levels before the biopsy. The patient must be kept NPO. After the test, the patient should rest in bed for twelve to twenty-four hours. If the patient complains of increased pain, check the vital signs. With increased pain, there is a possibility of bleeding occurring. The patient will complain of abdominal pressure. The patient is assessed for bleeding, and the physician will order to check the HCT level every six hours. Assess the patient for *shock* and *pneumothorax*. The patients remain on light activity for every biopsy for about two weeks.

GASTROINTESTINAL INTUBATION

Gastrostomy Tube (G-Tube; PEG-Tube)- Nasogastric Tube (NG-Tube)

A nasogastric tube is a thin, flexible plastic tube used for tube feeding, medication administration, and gastric suction. It is designed to pass through the nose, throat, and esophagus and into the stomach. Enteral nutrition is needed when the patient has difficulty swallowing (dysphagia) or has a type of cancer that interrupts nutrition. Nasogastric tubes may be single or double-lumen, depending on their need. When inserting the tube, assess for a deviated septum. Some facilities may have specific staff to insert these tubes.

Nursing Care

Assess placement before using the tube. This is done through a chest x-ray or by aspirating stomach content and testing its pH level. Patients must be sitting up during nutrition administration. After medication administration or feedings, irrigate/flush the tube. Verify that the medications being administered can be crushed. If not, request the physician to change them to a liquid form. Do not mix medications. Each medication should be given by itself. Dissolve medications in approximately ten to twenty ml of water and flush after. The physician will order frequent flushes throughout the day to check the patency of the tube.

After the first feeding, it is usual for the patients to experience liquid stools. If the patient experiences diarrhea every time, complains of nausea, and the nurse observes abdominal distention, the feeding must be turned off, and the physician and the dietitian must be notified. Some facilities do not conduct residual assessments. However, if the facility assesses residual, any residual >150ml might indicate possible obstruction. Assess daily weight.

NASOGASTRIC TUBES (NG) for GASTRIC DECOMPRESSION

Levine and Dobhoff Tubes

These single-lumen tubes are the most common and are used for intermittent suction to prevent nausea, vomiting, and distension after surgery. The Dobhoff tube has a weight on the end, which the Levine tube does not.

Nursing Care

Mouth and nares care is a critical assessment that must be conducted during every shift. Assess patency. The physician may order routine or more frequent evaluation of electrolytes and Arterial Blood Gases (ABGs). Irrigation should be done with NS unless the physician orders water. The use of NS is recommended because potassium and sodium can be depleted when water is used.

Salem Sump Tube

This is a double-lumen tube with an air vent used for continuous suction. One lumen is wider and used for suction, while the narrower lumen acts as a vent to relieve pressure from the vacuum. Reducing the pressure prevents the tube from adhering to the stomach. Its use and care are the same as those of the Levine tube.

DISORDERS OF THE GASTROINTESTINAL SYSTEM

Appendicitis and Peritonitis

Appendicitis is the inflammation of the appendix. The appendix is a pouch extending from the colon to where the small intestine empties its contents. This finger-like pouch is localized on the right lower quadrant of the abdomen. Appendicitis is caused by a blockage in the lining of the appendix. The appendix becomes inflamed relatively fast, with bacteria and other pathogens becoming infected. Signs and symptoms include acute pain, usually on the right lower quadrant and sometimes around the navel. Other symptoms include nausea and vomiting, loss of appetite, fever that may worsen as the illness progresses, constipation or diarrhea, abdominal bloating, and flatulence. Appendicitis is diagnosed by applying pressure to the site. When the pressure is released, the pain usually becomes worse. A ruptured appendix is a severe complication that requires surgery and the placement of a drain to remove pus.

Peritonitis is the inflammation of the peritoneum, the smooth tissue surrounding the abdominal organs and lining the abdominopelvic cavity. Perforation of the stomach, gallbladder, or lacerated liver could open the normally sterile peritoneum environment to microorganisms and pathogens, developing an inflammatory process. Multiple diagnostic tests, such as CT scans, X-rays, and laboratory tests, will help diagnose this condition. Strong antibiotics will be ordered to prevent the progression of the infection and the development of generalized sepsis.

Gastrointestinal Bleeding

Gastrointestinal bleeding can be observed in *emesis* (hematemesis) or melena (blood in stool). Depending on the facility's policy, the nurse may conduct a *hematest* with or without an order.

Gastroenteritis

This term is used to describe gastrointestinal alterations. Manifestation of this condition is related to the causative agent, but the presentation is usually diarrhea, vomiting, headache, fever, abdominal pain, and chills. Causative agents include *Clostridium difficile*, norovirus, and *Salmonella*. The infection occurs due to increased and continuous use of strong antibiotics, which reduces the normal flora and makes the patient susceptible to disease. If the manifestation of this condition worsens, the patient will have a deficit in electrolytes and fluids, putting the patient in a life-threatening situation. These microorganisms live in feces. The spread of these pathogens is through contaminated surfaces and the ingestion of contaminated food and water. Possible complications include perforation of the colon and sepsis.

Stress Ulcers

When under stress, the body produces sugar hormones like prednisone to cope. These hormones can lead to ulcers that damage the stomach lining. These ulcers may develop from trauma, septic shock, or other chronic conditions.

INTUSSUSCEPTION

Intussusception is when part of the intestine slides inside the adjacent intestines, resulting in obstruction of food, fluids, and blood, ischemia, and necrosis. Intussusception is rare in adults and most common in infants and children between six and eighteen years. Signs and symptoms are bowel obstruction and abdominal pain. This condition is an emergency and, left untreated, will be fatal in a few days. For infants and children, the treatment is therapeutic enemas. Surgery is the appropriate treatment for adults, often done laparoscopically.

DISORDERS OF THE GALLBLADDER

Cholecystitis/Cholelithiasis

Cholecystitis is gallbladder inflammation, and cholelithiasis is the formation of gallstones. Gallstones are hardened deposits of cholesterol/digestive fluid. Signs and symptoms are right upper quadrant (RUQ) pain, nausea, and vomiting, especially after consuming a high-cholesterol meal. Tests used to diagnose this condition are ultrasound, x-rays, and Endoscopic Retrograde Cholangiopancreatography (ERCP). The patient undergoes the same preparation for this test as for a gastroscopy. The treatment for this condition is surgery.

Nursing Care

Treat signs and symptoms. Pain management is essential for patients presenting this condition. It is important to remember that they should not receive morphine to alleviate the pain. Morphine causes spasms, and as a result, the pain level increases. Encourage fluid intake and change to a low-fat diet.

Cholecystectomy

This is the surgical removal of the gallbladder. It is a standard procedure that can also be performed laparoscopically with minimal invasion. After a chole-laparoscopy, the patient will experience right shoulder pain. To minimize the pain, the patient must be encouraged to ambulate.

DISORDERS OF THE PANCREAS

Pancreatitis

This is the inflammation of the pancreas. Signs and symptoms include left upper quadrant (LUQ) pain, nausea, and vomiting. It is diagnosed through ultrasound, enzyme levels, and blood glucose. An elevated Lipase level indicates a pancreatic problem. Insulin is produced in the pancreas, and the patient will experience an insulin deficiency. That is why these patients will have elevated blood glucose (hyperglycemia). The WBCs and the Calcium will also be elevated, but the HCT will be decreased. If the condition is critical, the physician may order a *pancreatography.* For a pancreatography, the patient will receive iodine dye. It is essential to assess the patient for possible allergy to iodine.

A complication of pancreatitis is shock due to hemorrhage. Nurses must assess Cullen's sign. Cullen's sign is the development of severe bruises that are reddish/purple spots around the belly button. This discoloration, called the Turner's sign, can also be seen over the kidneys' flanks. This is a sign that the pancreas is bleeding.

Nursing Care

The patient should be NPO (Nothing By Mouth). The physician will order Total Parenteral Nutrition (TPN). These patients should not receive morphine. The assessment should include Cullen's and Tuner's signs.

Total Parenteral Nutrition (TPN)

Total Parenteral Nutrition (TPN) is a feeding given through a vein, bypassing the gastrointestinal tract. The patient receives all the nutrients needed for the body to function well. A patient on TPN will often require a daily weight and chemistry profile. Blood glucose should also be monitored. The tubing should be changed every twenty-four hours because the nutrition will include lipids and glucose. The positioning of the patient is essential to prevent air embolism.

GASTROINTESTINAL CANCER

Cancer is the uncontrollable multiplication of abnormal cells forming a cluster of cells or tumors that intervene and affect the organ functionality. It develops its circulatory system.

Esophageal Cancer

Risk factors include alcohol, smoking, obesity, HPV, history of cancer, and age. This is common in elderly patients. This type of cancer is aggressive and does not show symptoms until it has spread. Symptoms include heartburn, pain in the throat, weight loss, chronic cough, vomiting or coughing up blood.

Colon Cancer

Risk factors include a history of rectal polyps, a family history of Inflammatory Bowel Disorder (IBD), smoked food intake, a low fiber diet, smoking, alcohol, processed food, obesity, and a high fat and beef protein diet. It is typically found in people 50 years of age and older, although recently it has been diagnosed in people 20 to 49. This type of cancer usually develops from polyps. Symptoms include melena (bloody stool), constipation, abdominal pain, bloated stomach, weight loss, anemia, and vomiting.

Oral Cancer

Risk factors include smoking, tobacco use, sun exposure (lip), HPV, and alcohol, affecting people 60 years of age and older. The person will develop white patches or bleeding sores. Other symptoms include weight loss, earache, chronic bad breath, numbness and pain in the face, and difficulty chewing or swallowing. There are different types of surgeries used to treat this cancer, depending on the stage. Chemotherapy, radiation therapy, immunotherapy, and the use of monoclonal antibodies are also treatment modalities used for this cancer.

Gastric/Stomach Cancer

Risk factors include a history of polyps, ulcers, pernicious anemia, smoking, and pickled food. It is most often found in people 65 years and older. Other causes include Helicobacter Pylori (H. pylori) infection, gastritis, GERD, Epstein-Barr virus infection, smoking, vaping, alcohol, obesity, and diet. There are also genetic conditions associated with gastric cancer. Although it can develop in any part of the stomach, it usually starts in the esophageal junction, where the esophagus meets the stomach. Symptoms include abdominal pain, difficulty swallowing, heartburn, indigestion, nausea and vomiting, weight loss, fatigue, black stools, and not feeling hungry or feeling full after a small meal.

Rectal Cancer

Risk factors include age, history of rectal polyps, family history of IBD, a history of *H. Pylori*, smoked food intake, a diet high in fat and beef protein, smoking, eating processed food, and obesity. Symptoms include rectal bleeding and changes in the frequency of bowel movements, diarrhea, constipation, weakness, abdominal pain, weight loss, and stool that is thin (like a pencil). Treatment includes surgery, chemotherapy, radiotherapy, and immunotherapy.

*Dark green vegetables, soy intake, and a glass of red wine a week protect the colon.

ESOPHAGEAL VARICES

When the liver has too much blood, the body develops collateral circulation, sending blood into the esophagus. Esophageal varices are also caused by alcohol intake and liver cirrhosis. The veins burst, and the patient starts to bleed. The main sign is a massive gastrointestinal bleed. The patient has difficulty clotting. The treatment includes placing a *Sengstacke–Blakemore tube* (S-B Tube).

The Sengstacke–Blakemore tube (S-B Tube) is a triple-lumen tube that stops bleeding in the esophagus. One lumen inflates the esophageal balloon, preventing blood from entering the stomach. The third lumen suctions blood from the stomach.

Nursing Care

The patients should be assessed for respiratory distress. If they are, the tube should be ~~is~~ cut to deflate the balloon.

HIATAL HERNIA and GASTROESOPHAGEAL REFLUX DISEASE (GERD)

Hiatal hernia results from a weakened muscle or tissue, allowing organs from the gastrointestinal system to bulge up through the *diaphragm.* The diaphragm is the muscle that separates the abdominal cavity from the chest cavity. The reason why this occurs is still being determined. The signs and symptoms include heartburn or acid reflux (GERD). Patients also complain of bloating, nausea, and vomiting.

Nursing Care

Patients are educated on the best diet they should ingest and to eat small, frequent meals. The physician will order antacids and histamine blockers, such as Cetirizine (Zyrtec), Hydroxyzine (Vistaril or Atarax), Diphenhydramine (Benadryl), Fexofenadine (Allegra), or Loratadine (Claritin). Education also includes avoiding lifting or bending and eating while sitting at ninety degrees and not before sleep. Patients should remain sitting for one to two hours after eating.

TRAUMA

Gastrointestinal injuries occur due to blunt force trauma, gunshot, or stabbing. Presentation, including signs and symptoms, depends on the degree of penetration and where the injury occurs. However, patients show altered mental status and consciousness due to blood loss. Hemorrhage may be visible, or it might occur internally. Patients will have tachycardia and hypotension to compensate for the loss of blood. Treatment is directed to restore and maintain fluid and volume balance. Nursing assessment is crucial to prevent infections. Depending on the extension of the traumatic injury, the patient will require surgery.

PEPTIC ULCER DISEASE

Gastric Ulcer

This condition is diagnosed through UGI and endoscopy. The patients complain of epigastric pain one to two hours after eating. A bacteria called *Helicobacter Pylori (H. Pylori*) causes ulcers in the stomach, with patients requiring antibiotics. This condition is a risk factor for cancer.

Nursing Care

The primary intervention is to assess pain and monitor diet. The patients are instructed to avoid food that irritates them and to eat frequently. Food relieves pain. When food does not reduce the pain, the stomach might be perforated.

Duodenal Ulcer

This is one of the more common ulcers. It is diagnosed the same way as the gastric ulcer. An increased secretion of acid in the stomach causes the development of this ulcer. The patients complain of pain two to four hours after eating, especially at night.

Nursing Care

Pain assessment and management are essential interventions. Offer the same diet education as for gastric ulcers. Anti-ulcer medications should be taken at night.

Anti-Ulcer Medications			
Medications	Action	Administration	Adverse Reactions
Histamine Antagonists "tidiness."	Inhibits gastric acid secretion by blocking histamine receptors on parietal cells.	Give Tagamet with meals. Please do not give it to elderly patients because it will confuse them. All other medications can be taken without food. Do not give Axid	Headaches

		with vegetable juices. Cautiously use Zantac in renal or liver disease patients.	
Proton Pump Inhibitors "prazoles"	Inhibits the proton (acid) pump needed to stimulate parietal cells to secrete gastric acid.	It can be taken without regard to meals. Give a daily dose at night. Use cautiously in renal or liver disease patients.	Headaches Cough Diarrhea

Antacids			
Medications	Action	Administration	Adverse Reactions
Aluminum "gels"	Neutralizes acid by elevating gastric pH to decrease acid activity. It also strengthens the mucosal barrier and increases esophageal sphincter tone, preventing reflux.	Separate administration from other drugs by one to two hours.	Constipation Aluminum toxicity
Calcium Carbonate	Same as above	Separate administration from other drugs by one to two hours. Alternate with Magnesium to prevent constipation	Constipation Hypercalcemia (causes kidney stones)

Antacids			
Medications	Action	Administration	Adverse Reactions
Magnesium	Same as above	Separate administration from other drugs by one to two hours. Alternate with Calcium Carbonate to prevent constipation	Diarrhea Hypermagnesemia

Combination Antacids Aluminum-Magnesium (Riopan)			
Medications	Action	Administration	Adverse Reactions
Mucosal Barrier Protector (Sulcralfate=Carafate)	Provides a protective adhesive barrier around and over the ulcer	Take on an empty stomach one hour before meals and at bedtime. Separate administration from antacids by at least 30 minutes	Constipation

GASTRIC SURGERIES

Billroth I – Gastroduodenostomy (Stomach)

This is the removal of the lower portion of the stomach.

Billroth II -Gastrojejunostomy (Duodenum)

For this surgical procedure, the lower end of the stomach and the duodenum are removed and attached to the jejunum. This procedure is like bariatric surgery. The patient will be on a vitamin B-12 regimen for this procedure to prevent *pernicious anemia*. These patients are also at risk of *dumping syndrome.*

Dumping Syndrome (Rapid Gastric Emptying)

This condition occurs especially after stomach surgery, but it can also happen after esophagus surgery. After surgery, food high in sugar increases the peristalsis of the intestines, causing food to move too quickly from the stomach to the small intestine. Signs and symptoms are abdominal pain; the patient feels tired and needs to lie down. This can occur one to three hours after eating. The patient may experience vertigo, nausea, cramps, sweating, and vomiting.

Nursing Care

The patient should be encouraged to lie down after eating for approximately two hours. Meals should be small, frequent, and dry; liquids should be ingested between meals and not with meals.

DISEASES OF THE GASTROINTESTINAL SYSTEM

INFLAMMATORY BOWEL SYNDROME (IBS)

Immune response to the normal flora in the intestine results in a disease characterized by bowel inflammation. The areas affected most often are the ileum and the colon. There is a high incidence of colon cancer in patients with this condition. The treatment goal is attaining remission and prevention of recurrent attacks. Emergency care is focused on the prevention of hemorrhage and bowel obstruction.

Crohn's Disease

This is an autoimmune disease characterized by gastrointestinal system inflammation (IBD). There is a genetic predisposition for this condition. The patients will experience right lower quadrant (RLQ) pain, distention, fatigue, and severe diarrhea. This condition is diagnosed through a colonoscopy. This is a very debilitating condition. To avoid the signs and symptoms, the patients sometimes are malnourished. This condition can be treated with medication such as *Remicaid (Infliximab).* Remicaid is a monoclonal antibody used to treat autoimmune diseases.

Nursing Care

The patients should be educated on a low-residue, low-fiber diet. They should also avoid foods rich in carbohydrates that produce gas, such as broccoli, onions, potatoes, and cauliflower. Administer anti-diarrheal medication and provide pain management.

Ulcerative Colitis

This is one of the worst gastrointestinal conditions. Like Crohn's disease, ulcerative colitis is an autoimmune condition characterized by bowel inflammation. However, this condition develops ulcers in the colon and rectum. It presents with abdominal pain, cramps, rectal bleeding, and bloody stools. The patient will also have weight loss. This condition is diagnosed by colonoscopy and biopsy. Patients are at risk for colon cancer.

Nursing Care

Patients with this condition might be placed on TPN. The diet should be low-fiber and low-residue. Pain management and peri-anal care are the primary interventions.

Diverticulosis/Diverticulitis

Diverticulosis is the development of weak areas on the intestine wall that break, forming bulging pouches. When those pouches become inflamed, it is called diverticulitis. Patients complain of intermittent pain in the left lower quadrant (LLQ) and have episodes of constipation and diarrhea. Diagnosis is done through a colonoscopy and LGI.

Nursing Care

Patients are put on TPN. Regular meals are modified to high fiber and low *roughage* diet. Roughage is fiber the body cannot digest. This fiber can be found in nuts, seeds, whole grains, and legumes. The physician will order bulk laxatives.

OSTOMIES

Ostomies are surgically created openings on the abdomen that help remove waste from the body. It brings a section of the intestine/colon through the abdominal wall. The opening is called a *stoma*. The location of the opening determines the consistency of the stools. The pouch should have gas after the surgery. This is indicative that the intestine is working. The higher the ostomy, the more liquid the stools will be. Ostomies can be temporary or permanent. The location specifies the types of ostomies.

Colostomy

An ostomy created on the *ascending* colon will cause bowel movements that are pasty and loose. The stoma will be located on the right side of the abdomen. A colonoscopy created in the *descending* colon will have soft and formed stools. The stoma will be located on the left side of the abdomen. This is the only opening that can be irrigated.

Nursing Care

The stoma should be pink, red, moist, and no bleeding. Keep the stoma dry. Perform frequent skin assessments. Monitor the patients for depression. Ostomies create self-esteem disturbance due to altered image disturbance. Please only force the patient to see it if they are ready.

DISORDERS OF THE LIVER

Diagnostic Tests

Liver Biopsy

Invasive procedure. Aspiration/Removal of a liver sample.

Alanine Aminotransferase (ALT)

Liver enzyme. Blood test. Normal value <35

Aspartate Aminotransferase (AST)

The liver enzyme is found when there is liver damage. Blood test. Normal value <40

Ammonia Level

This blood test will be elevated when patients present an altered mental status.

Albumin

Blood test. Normal value >6. If the patient has a liver disease, this test will be <6.

Alkaline Phosphatase

Blood test. This enzyme helps diagnose liver, bone, or kidney disease. Depending on the laboratory, the expected value range can be between thirty and one hundred and twenty IU/L.

PT/INR

In liver disease, these tests will be elevated.

Hepatitis – Types A, B, and C

Hepatitis viruses attack the liver, and it becomes inflamed. High alcohol consumption, toxins, and medications can cause it. It can also be autoimmune hepatitis. This is more dangerous.

Stage I – Flu-like symptoms, *pre-jaundice*

Stage II – Severe flu-like symptoms and *jaundice*

Stage III – Recovery

Hepatitis Panel (Hepatitis Antigen and Antibodies Tests): This is the blood test done for hepatitis. It can tell if the patient has had hepatitis or received the vaccine.

Hepatitis A

Hepatitis A appears when the patient has consumed food or water and is infected with fecal matter. It can happen when people do not wash their hands after using the bathroom or frequent public pools. People can recover on their own with no lasting damage to the liver.

Hepatitis B

This type occurs when people are exposed to body fluids, share needles, or engage in sex with an infected individual. People can recover with no lasting damage to the liver; however, some may remain with a chronic hepatitis infection that can lead to liver cancer.

Hepatitis C

Hepatitis C is the result of a person being exposed to infected blood. People remain with a long-lasting infection even after receiving medication. If not treated, this type can lead to cirrhosis of the liver and liver cancer.

Nursing Care

A sign of liver damage is the patient developing a "liver flap" or asterixis. This is the involuntary flexion of the hand, especially when the patient tries to extend the wrist. It simulates a bird flapping its wings. Standard precautions should be taken for all types. Patients are kept on bed rest with no visitors. It is recommended that patients consume five to seven small frequent meals. The diet should be high in protein, high in vitamins, and high in carbohydrates. Ammonia level might be elevated. If the level continues to increase, the patients will become confused. A diet low in protein is essential for patients with an elevated ammonia level. If the protein is not restricted, the patient will develop hepatic encephalopathy with a life expectancy of nine months to one year.

Fetor hepaticus, also known as "the breath of the dead," is a sign of hepatic encephalopathy. It is different from bad breath. Fetor hepaticus is a chronic condition indicating liver damage, as the liver is not processing toxins correctly.

Antiemetics should be given before eating. Compazine should NOT be used because it will make the jaundice worse. Skincare is essential. Patients will feel their skin itching. It is recommended that they use warm water and oatmeal baths.

Cirrhosis of the Liver

Cirrhosis is like hepatitis, with the patient developing ascites. It appears in patients diagnosed with Hepatitis B or C, but it is most prevalent in patients with Hepatitis C. Tests include a liver panel, PT, CBC, and ammonia level.

This condition is treated with vitamins, *lactulose*, and albumin administration. Lactulose is a medication that helps prevent ammonia from being absorbed into the system. This medication will cause the patient to have two to three soft stools.

Nursing Care

Encourage bed rest and a diet like the one for patients with hepatitis. Protein intake should be moderate to high in protein unless the ammonia level is high. Skincare is essential. Provide lotions to cool the skin and reduce the itching. Daily weights are necessary to determine if the patient is retaining fluids. Encourage the use of abdominal girth.

Ascites

Ascites is a condition characterized by abnormal fluid retention in the abdominal cavity. Ascites develops because the body is not producing enough albumin or not producing it at all. When the albumin level is decreased, water leaves the blood cells and builds up between the two layers that cover the peritoneum. The fluid can also surround the lungs, making it difficult to breathe. The patient will also develop pitting or peripheral edema on the lower extremities. The treatment consists of an invasive procedure called *paracentesis*.

Nursing Care

Follow the same diet/restrictions as the diet offered to patients with hepatitis. The diet must be low in sodium and low in protein. The dietitian will put the patient on fluid restriction. Conduct daily weights on the patient with ascites. This is the best indicator of the progression of the condition. Encourage the patients to wear abdominal girth. Educate the patients on the use of lactulose and the administration of albumin. Patients should remain in the *Hi-Fowler's* position to prevent *orthopnea*. Advise the patients to avoid the use of *Neomycin.* Neomycin is contraindicated because it is nephrotoxic.

CHAPTER 9 THE NERVOUS SYSTEM

The nervous system is integral to every action a person performs. It comprises three primary components: the brain, spinal cord, and nerves. This system is responsible for movement, thought, and sensation and autonomously manages processes such as digestion. It encompasses both the central and peripheral nervous systems.

DIAGNOSTIC TESTS

Brain Scan CT scan

A computerized tomography scan uses X-rays to take pictures of the brain and surrounding area. If patients experience headaches or other symptoms or the physician is concerned, a brain scan is one of the first imaging tests ordered.

Nursing Care

Before the test, the nurse assesses the patient for dye allergies. The patient must remain still to ensure the pictures come out correctly. After the test, the nurse instructs the patient to increase their fluid intake.

Lumbar Puncture (Spinal Tap)

This test removes a cerebrospinal fluid (CSF) sample surrounding the brain and spinal cord. It is used to diagnose infections, diseases, bleeding, and cancer.

Nursing Care

Assist the physician by positioning the patient correctly. The patient should be in the fetal position. Sometimes, the patient sits on the edge of the bed and leans over the table. This position helps to open the vertebrae and facilitates needle insertion. After the procedure, the patient must remain flat and supine in bed for several hours. This is important to prevent the patient from developing excruciating headaches. Headaches after this procedure are an indication of leakage of the CSF.

Cerebral Angiogram/Angiography

A cerebral angiogram uses X-rays to visualize the inside of the blood vessels. This test helps identify brain bleeds, aneurysms, abnormalities, or clots. A thin catheter is placed in an artery that travels to the brain. The dye is administered, and pictures are taken. When the catheter is inserted, plaque or thrombus inside the artery may be dislodged, putting the patient at risk for stroke.

Nursing Care

Before the test, assess the patient for dye allergies. Peripheral pulses and vital signs must be evaluated before and after the test. Encourage the patient to increase fluid intake. The patient should remain in bed for up to six hours and then ambulate.

Electroencephalogram (EEG)

This test assesses brain activity and helps identify and diagnose disorders like epilepsy.

Nursing Care

Educate the patient to wash their hair the night before and not use creams or conditioners. The patient may need to be asleep during the test, so they should be instructed not to sleep or sleep less the night before. Before starting the test, the patient should avoid ingesting coffee, tea, or chocolate.

Magnetic Resonance Imaging (MRI)

This imaging technique uses magnetic fields and computer-generated radio waves to create detailed images of organs and tissues inside the body.

Nursing Care

Assess the patient for metal in the body, including tattoos. Patients with tattoos undergoing this test will see the tattoo inflamed and swollen. Also, the patient should be asked if the individual is claustrophobic or if the patient is afraid of noise. Some patients will require the use of antianxiety medication.

DISORDERS OF THE NEUROSENSORY SYSTEM

Increased Intracranial Pressure (ICP)

After trauma, aneurysm, tumor, stroke, bleeding, or brain lesion, the intracranial pressure may become elevated. The first sign will be a headache. This is a critical emergency because the increased pressure can further damage the brain. Besides the headache, the patient can complain of blurred vision, sleepiness, difficulty moving the extremities, and vomiting.

Other signs and symptoms include decreased *consciousness (LOC),* apical pulse, respirations, and widening pulse pressure. Widening of the pulse pressure will be evident by an increase in the systolic BP. For example, the BP will change from 120/80 with a pulse pressure of 40 to 150/80 with a pulse pressure of 70. Another symptom is an elevated temperature. Because of the intracranial pressure, the *hypothalamus* is not working, and the patient will develop increased temperature. The hypothalamus is deep inside the brain, connecting the endocrine and nervous systems. This tiny structure maintains *homeostasis* (balance) in the body, regulating pulse and temperature, among other things. Increased Intracranial Pressure (ICP) is diagnosed through a CT scan.

Nursing Care

Position the patient in a low Fowler's position. If the patient is unconscious, position the patient in low Fowler's lateral position. The patient should not be placed for hip flexion. Legs should remain extended. Assess the airway first. Check the amount of fluids consumed, LOC, and vital signs. Assess the patient for a CSF leak. Check the CSF for sugar.

Medications that might be administered are Mannitol (diuretic), steroids (to reduce inflammation), stool softeners, Valium, Tagamet (to prevent stress ulcers), and muscle relaxants.

Continue monitoring the ICP to keep it <15mmHG. Conduct a *Glasgow Coma Scale (GCS).*

Glasgow Coma Scale (GCS)

The Glasgow Coma Scale (GCS) assesses patients' consciousness in three areas of responsiveness: eye-opening (E), motor (M), and verbal responses (V). Use the GCS every time patients experience acute medical or trauma impairment. Document a GCS of eight as E2V3M3. If the GCS is <12, the patient's condition is terrible. If the GCS is < 8, the patient's condition is worse.

GLASGOW COMA SCALE (0-15)			
Eye Response	1.	No eye opening	*Best Score*
	2.	Eye-opening to pain	*4*
	3.	Eye-opening to sound	
	4.	Eyes open spontaneously	
Verbal Response	1.	No verbal response	*Best Score*
	2.	Incomprehensible sounds	*5*
	3.	Inappropriate words	
	4.	Confused	
	5.	Orientated	
Motor Response	1.	No motor response.	*Best Score*
	2.	Abnormal extension to pain	*6*
	3.	Abnormal flexion to pain	
	4.	Withdrawal from pain	
	5.	Localizing pain	
	6.	Obey commands	

Brain Death

A negative EEG for brain activity will diagnose a patient brain dead. Signs and Symptoms include the *doll's eyes.* In the doll's eyes, the patient's eyes stay fixed when the head is turned. Another test performed on patients suspected of brain death is the *caloric test.* This test involves using cold water inside the ear canal and changing the temperature. This will produce rapid side-to-side eye movement. This will not occur in a patient that is brain dead.

Medications include Mannitol (diuretic), steroids (to reduce inflammation), stool softeners, valium and muscle relaxants, and Tagamet (to prevent stress ulcers).

Nursing Care

The first step when conducting patient assessment is checking the airway. Fluids for these patients are contraindicated. Assess the LOC and vital signs. Another critical assessment is CSF leaks. If the wipe turns yellow, it is CSF. Check for sugar in the CSF. Check for sugar in the CSF. Keep the legs of brain-dead patients extended, never hip flexion. The nurse monitors for ICP. Intracranial pressure is kept <15 mmHG. The GCS goal is > 9. The best position for an unconscious patient is on a side low Fowler's.

Intracranial Surgery (Craniotomy)

The patient will present a *supratentorial or infratentorial incision*. The supratentorial incision has the letter "C" upside down. The infratentorial incision also has the letter "C" upside down but on the back portion of the skull. Maintain the patient flat in bed. Check vital signs every hour. Assess the temperature to determine if there is damage to the hypothalamus. Monitor urine output.

COMPLICATIONS OF INCREASED INTRACRANIAL PRESSURE

Hyperthermia

Hyperthermia results from hypothalamus malfunction. Keep the patient warm, but do not provide fluids to prevent the ICP from increasing.

Syndrome of inappropriate antidiuretic hormone ADH release (SIADH)

The syndrome of inappropriate antidiuretic hormone (ADH) release (SIADH) occurs due to malignancies or CNS disturbances. The antidiuretic hormone (ADH) is responsible for the water balance in the system. In SIADH, a sign is a fluid overload. The pituitary secretes ADH. Complications from the pituitary gland can cause SIADH. Other causes are drugs, surgeries, pulmonary disease, hormone deficiency, hormone administration, HIV, or hereditary SIADH.

The level of ADH is high in patients with SIADH, causing hyponatremia. The sodium level drops as low as 125-130 mEq/L, causing headaches, vomiting, nausea, confusion, problems with ambulation, memory, and cognitive issues. The sodium in urine will be >40mEq/L. Treatment is the use of diuretics.

Diabetes Insipidus

A decreased secretion of ADH causes diabetes insipidus. Signs and symptoms include hypovolemia presented by *polyuria* (urine output >200ml/hr.) for two hours, decreased specific gravity, reduced urine osmolality, and increased serum osmolality. The first assessment the physician does when a suspicion of diabetes insipidus exists is checking the specific gravity. Treatment includes the use of desmopressin acetate (DDAVP).

CEREBRAL VASCULAR ACCIDENTS (CVA)

Another name for CVA is *Stroke* because it strikes the patient when the cerebral perfusion or blood circulation is blocked. Hypertension, illicit drug abuse, *atherosclerotic heart disease* (ASHD), diabetes mellitus vascular changes, and clotting disorders are the leading causes of CVA.

Types

Hemorrhagic Stroke

For this type, nothing is to be done.

Thrombolytic/Thrombosis/Ischemic Stroke

For this type, thrombolytic agents are given. Tissue plasminogen activator (tPA) is the ideal medication to be administered. This medication removes all the clotting factors within five hours after a CVA. This medication restores circulation in the affected part of the brain before it is dead.

Signs and symptoms include headaches, HTN, increased respirations, altered LOC, weakness, incontinence, *dysarthria* (difficulty speaking), *aphasia* (loss of the ability to understand or express speech), *and apraxia* (the patient cannot move). Diagnosis is through a brain CT scan. The physician may order a *transesophageal echocardiogram* (TEE) to identify the source of the clot.

Nursing Care

Airway assessment and vital signs are the first interventions. These patients are at risk for orthostatic hypotension after bed rest. Place the patient on the side in a low Fowler's position. Patients who experience a CVA, depending on the area in the brain where the CVA occurs, may present expressive or receptive aphasia. *Expressive aphasia* is the inability to speak or write to express themselves. In these patients, comprehension is intact. Patients become frustrated because they cannot make themselves understood. *Receptive aphasia* is the inability to understand what is being said to them. This condition is like taking care of a baby.

Assess the patient's ability to eat by assessing the gag reflex. The patient may have an order to be evaluated by Speech Therapy. This is done by determining the patient's ability to swallow without choking. One way to assist the patient in eating is by massaging or tucking in the chin.

"The head is upright to receive a bite of food, the food is chewed and rotated in the mouth to form a bolus, before swallowing, the chin is dropped into a chin-tuck, and the swallow is initiated. This process is helpful for those with difficulty with lip closure and keeping food in their mouth while chewing" (Mealtime Partners, Inc., 2018).

Skin assessment and care are essential interventions for patients at risk for injury due to impaired mobility. A physical therapist will assess the patient and write recommendations or orders for *range of motion* (ROM) exercises. A range of motion exercises help maintain the patient's mobility and prevents contractures from developing. Elimination is essential to avoid constipation or fecal impaction.

Homonymous Hemianopia (Hemianopsia)

In this condition, the visual field is compromised, presenting blindness in each eye on the paralyzed side of the body. Nursing intervention involves teaching patients to scan the environment to prevent falls and injuries.

Transient Ischemic Attack (TIA)

This is a temporary impairment of cerebral blood flow. It is usually identified by vision impairment or the patient becoming nonresponsive. Treatments include ASA (Aspirin), Heparin, and other anticoagulation medications *("blood thinners").* The physician may order a *carotid endarterectomy* only if the patient's life expectancy is in jeopardy. Carotid Endarterectomy removes plaque or fatty deposits built up in the arteries, specifically the carotid arteries.

SPINAL CORD INJURY (SCI)

The spinal cord is the structure that connects the brainstem to the body, carrying nerve signals back and forth between the brain and the rest of the body. Any damage or trauma that disrupts the communication between the brain and the body will result in *paralysis*. Paralysis is the inability to move parts of the body. The mobility impairment will be more extensive depending on the injury's location. *Quadriplegia* is a paralysis from the neck down that occurs when the spinal cord injury (SCI) occurs to the cervical spine (C-Spine). If the injury occurs in the lower part of the spinal cord, the patient will not be able to move their legs. This is called *paraplegia.* There are different types of paralysis.

Quadriplegia

The muscles will act in two different ways when the patient develops quadriplegia: *flaccid* or *spastic.* Flaccid muscles will not work, remaining flaccid all the time. Spastic muscles will contract uncontrollably.

Incomplete Quadriplegia

The injury blocks some but not all the nerve signals. The patient will experience some sensations and might be able to experience and control some bladder and bowel functions.

Complete Quadriplegia

The injury blocks all the nerve signals from the brain to the body. Complete quadriplegia affects C1-C2. The patient will lose control of movement. The patient will not be able to ambulate or have sensations from the neck down. This injury can be fatal if not treated on time. The patient will have difficulty breathing because it cuts communication with the *autonomic nervous system*. The autonomic nervous system controls all the automatic responses and functions in the body, such as sweating, blood pressure control, digestion, and the muscles that control the bladder and bowels.

When the injury involves C3-C4, the patients will have difficulty breathing and coughing. These patients are at risk for pneumonia and must be repositioned often. For injury involving C4-C7, the patient will have some paralysis in the arms.

Nursing Care

Nursing interventions should be implemented immediately. The airway is the first area to be assessed. Determine if the patient is experiencing *spinal shock.*

Spinal shock is the term used to describe when the patient is experiencing flaccidity and rigidity in the muscles and cannot have reflexes. Identify if the patient developed *autonomic dysreflexia (hyperreflexia).* Patients often require the insertion of an NGT. Repositioning is essential for these patients to prevent pneumonia and pressure injuries from occurring. Assess skin frequently. These patients will be receiving steroids to decrease the inflammation.

Regarding elimination, if the patient has *upper SCI, the muscles that control the* bowels and bladder will be spastic and will need stimulation. To assist with urination, the nurse will apply *Crede's maneuver. Crede's maneuver* is a technique where pressure is applied over the abdomen, the bladder area, and below the navel. Patients will require the use of suppositories to assist with bowel movements. If the patient has a *lower SCI,* the patient will need to be straight catheterized, usually every six hours. These patients will also require manual decompaction to prevent bowel obstruction.

AUTONOMIC DYSREFLEXIA (HYPERREFLEXIA)

When the thoracic nerves are involved in a spinal cord injury (>T6), the patient will experience a sudden elevation in blood pressure. This syndrome is called autonomic dysreflexia, and it is a life-threatening condition. The main sign and symptom of this condition is headache. Other signs and symptoms besides headache are goose flesh above the level of the injury, diaphoresis, nausea, blurred vision, high BP, and bradycardia. Autonomic dysreflexia usually occurs after a n*eurogenic shock* has resolved.

The primary nursing intervention is to immediately place the patient in a semi-fowler's position and assess the immediate environment for stimulating factors. A stimulus can trigger the autonomic dysreflexia response, affecting the bladder, the bowels, and the skin. Therefore, the nurse must assess the bladder, Foley catheter, and rectum. The nurse must check bladder drainage and restore it if it is blocked. The same should be done when checking the Foley catheter for any blockage or malfunction. Testing the urine for a possible urinary tract infection (UTI) is necessary. A rectal exam is required to prevent fecal impaction or to perform decompactions.

Neurogenic Shock

Patients with SCI >T6 develop a syndrome called neurogenic shock. This condition prevents the body from regulating vital signs, especially blood pressure, heart rate, and temperature. The body does not receive a signal to constrict the blood vessels, so they remain in vasodilation (vessels open too much), lowering the blood pressure. This is dangerous because it prevents oxygen from reaching the organs.

DISEASES OF THE NEUROLOGIC SYSTEM

MULTIPLE SCLEROSIS (MS)

Another name used for this disease is *demyelination disease*. This name describes what occurs in MS. The myelin sheath that covers and protects the nerves is damaged and destroyed, interrupting the communication between the brain and the body. As the disease progresses, patients' mobility will be compromised, with MS patients losing the ability to ambulate. The patients will complain of vision problems *(nystagmus),* temporary blindness, muscle weakness, paresthesia, and *neurogenic bladder*.

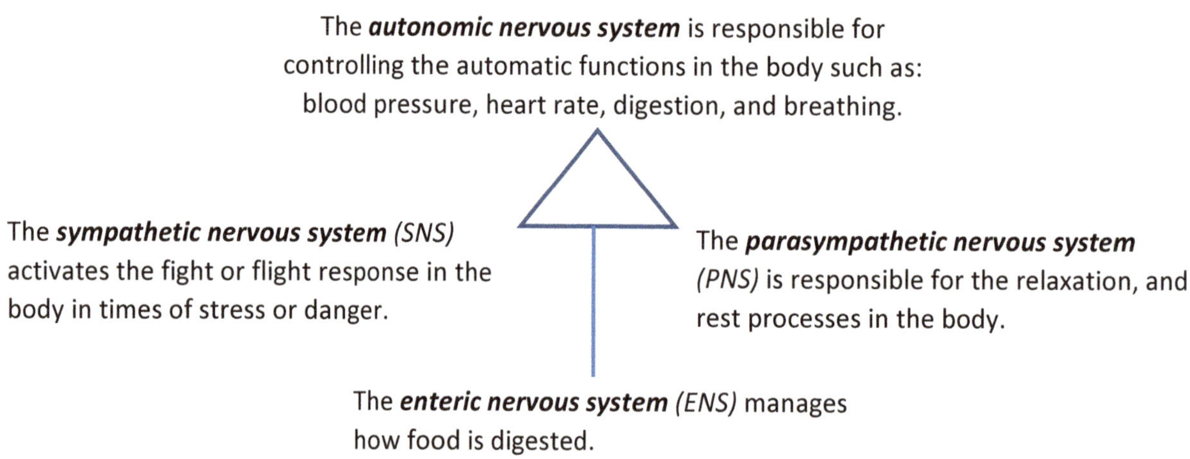

Multiple Sclerosis progresses slowly. Diagnostic tests used are Electromyograms (EMG), which measure a muscle's electrical activity, and MRIs, which show demyelinated areas in the brain. Medications and therapies ordered are Methotrexate (MTX), Interferon B, steroids, and Valium.

Nursing Care

Patients must rest and avoid fatigue, infections, stress, and crowds. Their diet should be acidic to acidify the urine and fluids to prevent UTIs. Education on birth control is essential. Skin assessment and care daily for injuries related to paresthesia are also critical. Emotional support is also necessary.

MYASTHENIA GRAVIS (Severe Muscle Weakness)

A breakdown in the communication between the nerves and the muscles develops severe muscle weakness. This condition has no cure. Symptoms include *diplopia* (double vision), drooping eyelids, and difficulties with speech *(dysarthria*), chewing, swallowing (*dysphasia*), and breathing (*dyspnea*).

To diagnose myasthenia gravis, the patient is injected with *Tensilon* IV and is diagnosed positive if the patient regains muscle strength.

Nursing Care

Assess respiratory status and gag reflexes before meals. The diet is mechanical, soft, and thick liquids. Medications ordered include *Prostigmine, Mestinon*, and *Neostigmine*. These medications improve muscle strength by preventing the breakdown of *acetylcholine* in the body. Acetylcholine is a neurotransmitter needed for normal muscle function.

Myasthenia Crisis vs. Cholinergic Crisis		
	Myasthenia Crisis	Cholinergic Crisis
1. Cause	Not much *Tensilon* was administered	Too much *Tensilon* administered
2. Signs and Symptoms	Disease exacerbation presented by *increased drooling and muscle weakness*	S – Salivation L – Lacrimation U – Urination D – Defecation G – Gastric Issues E – Emesis
1. Results	Muscle strength returns caused by *under-medication*	Respiratory/Cardiac Arrest caused by *over-medication*
2. Treatment	Increased medication *(Tensilon)* dose	Administer *ATROPINE STAT* to reverse the effects of *Tensilon* and reduce the medication *(Tensilon)* dose.

PARKINSON'S DISEASE

Parkinson's Disease is a disease that affects the neurologic system and presents as incontrollable tremors. The cause is unknown, although some studies suggest it is related to *Dopamine* deficiency. Dopamine is a neurotransmitter used by the nerve cells to communicate. Another possible reason is environmental and is associated with carbon monoxide or manganese poisoning. Symptoms start slowly. The patient's mobility will be compromised because the disease can cause stiffness. As the disease progresses, signs and symptoms will become more disturbing. A classic sign is the *pill-rolling tremor*. The patient will rub the thumb and forefinger back and forth. Other signs and symptoms include *bradykinesia* (slow movement), which turns simple tasks into time-consuming tasks. Patients shuffle their feet, and their speech becomes monotone, slurred, and challenging to understand—automatic movements such as blinking, smiling, and swinging the arms when ambulating will decrease. The patient will have trouble writing, and the posture will become stooped. Parkinson's patients are at high risk for falls and respiratory problems. The rib cage will feel tight.

Medications prescribed include Sinemet (carbidopa/Levodopa). This medication crosses the blood-brain barrier, helping to control the tremors. A common side effect is orthostatic hypotension, urinary retention, and constipation, among other symptoms.

Nursing Care

Provide a safe environment for the patients, assess the skin often, and help meet psychological needs. Family members and friends can be a great support system for patients with this condition. Educate the family on ways to meet psychological needs.

Guillain-Barre Syndrome (Acute Infectious Polyneuritis)

This syndrome is an immune system disease that causes damage to the nerves. The cause is unknown; however, it is believed that a virus causes it. Patients diagnosed with COVID-19, Zika virus, or a respiratory or gastrointestinal infection report symptoms of an infection before being diagnosed with Guillain-Barre Syndrome. Patients will experience ascending *paralysis*. Treatments will help ease the symptoms, but severe cases can be fatal. The lasting effects include weakness, numbness, and fatigue. The patient will present respiratory acidosis. The complication is respiratory failure. EMG, lumbar puncture, and MRI tests diagnose Guillain-Barre Syndrome.

PARKINSON'S DISEASE=Dopamine deficiency causing stiffness, rigidity, and tremors

SAFETY

- Friction soles
- No clutter
- No rugs

DIET

- Mechanical soft
- Low protein
- Thick liquids

ACTIVITIES

- Marching stationary bicycling (Tandem walking=heel-toe marching)

MEDICATIONS

- Levodopa
- Sinemet

Nursing Care

Maintaining an open airway is the primary intervention for these patients. Educate the patients on the use of the *incentive spirometer*. Incentive spirometer exercises should be performed ten times every hour. They help expand the lungs and open the blood vessels to increase oxygen capacity, clear out mucus, strengthen the lungs, and lower the risk of lung infection after surgery.

Assess the patient for dysphagia and skin for prevention of pressure injuries, assist with *PROM* (Passive Range of Motion), and offer support to meet psychological needs, especially communication methods.

BELL'S PALSY

This is reversible facial paralysis. In this condition, the facial nerve is irritated, and one side *(unilateral)* of the face becomes paralyzed. The facial nerve (nerve 7) is in front of the ear. Patients who develop this condition have a history of herpes simplex/zoster (Shingles). Treatment includes anticonvulsant medications to decrease the excitability of the *neurons*. The neurons are the cells responsible for receiving the input from the environment in the neurologic system and passing it on to the muscles as an electrical signal.

Patients diagnosed with Bell's Palsy are often prescribed analgesics and anticonvulsants such as *Tegretol.*

Nursing Care

Educate the patients to avoid cold and heat, patch the affected eye, and use artificial tears. To exercise the face, the patients can practice chewing and smiling. Massaging the affected side of the face with upward motion can also help ease the symptoms.

DISEASE AND DISORDERS OF THE EYE

Detached Retina

The retina is a tissue connected at the back of the eye that reacts to light. The light triggers electrical impulses that pass through the optical nerve to the brain, forming the visual image. The retinal detachment is not painful, but the signs and symptoms should be addressed quickly to prevent or reduce the risk of permanent vision loss. When the retina detaches, the tissue stops receiving blood and oxygen. Signs and symptoms include decreased vision, flashes of light, floaters in the visual field, and progressive vision loss. Treatment is surgery, and the patient will go blind if untreated.

Nursing Care

Before surgery, patch both eyes, maintain the patient on bed rest, and increase safety measures to prevent falls and injuries, using the backs of chairs and armrests as support (dependent position). After surgery, patch the affected eye and maintain light activity. Continue using the dependent position.

Glaucoma

Glaucoma is the damage to the optic nerve caused by increased pressure in the eye. However, it can occur with normal eye pressure. It can happen at any age but is more common in older adults. Signs and symptoms include decreased peripheral vision, HALOS around the objects, and *mydriasis* (dilation of the pupils). The patients will require surgery (*Trabeculectomy*) to relieve aqueous *humor fluid* (clear liquid or gel inside the front of the eye, keeping it inflated).

Nursing Care

Prescription eye drops and stool softeners will be ordered. Patients should avoid bending over and be careful when coughing or emesis. It is essential not to use Valsalva's maneuver, a breathing technique used to decelerate the heart rate in some arrhythmias and increase blood pressure in other areas, such as the inner ears and sinuses.

Cataracts (Clouds)

Aging and long-term use of steroids are risk factors for cataracts. The main signs and symptoms are the development of a "cloud" over the lens and decreased vision or blindness. Treatment is surgery, the implantation of Intraocular Cataract Lenses (IOLs).

Nursing Care

Patients who suffer from cataracts are at high risk for falls and injuries. They become afraid and have the potential for social isolation. The primary nursing intervention is to maintain the patient safe and prevent falls and injuries. Before surgery, the *ciliary muscle* paralyzes. The ciliary muscle is the muscle responsible for the accommodation of the eye to capture objects at different distances. It also regulates the aqueous fluid in the eye. After the surgery, the patient should avoid driving for at least three months until vision is restored.

Xerosis

Xerosis is the dryness of the skin, mucous membranes (*xerostomia*-dry mouth), or conjunctiva (*xerophthalmia*-dry eyes).

DISEASE OF THE EAR

Meniere's Disease

Meniere's disease is a rare condition of the inner ear, causing *vertigo* and the sensation of spinning. Vertigo is a type of dizziness that requires medical attention. There are two types of vertigo. There are many reasons for vertigo to appear, but problems with the inner ear most likely cause it. This is called peripheral vertigo. The second type of vertigo is called central vertigo and is associated with traumatic brain injuries and stroke. Meniere's disease has no cause or cure but is associated with sodium intake. Signs and symptoms include loss of hearing (a sensorineural hearing loss) that can be unilateral or bilateral. Treatment consists of a low sodium diet, decreasing the fluid in the middle ear. Patients will be prescribed Antivert or Dramamine and scopolamine patches. Ginger is also recommended to prevent nausea. Patients are encouraged to maintain a quiet, non-stimulating environment (low light).

BRAIN STRUCTURES AND FUNCTIONS

Brainstem - connects the brain to the spinal cord. It is located at the bottom of the brain and includes the *midbrain, pons, and medulla oblongata.* The brainstem sends messages to the rest of the body to regulate balance, breathing, and heart rate, among other things.

Midbrain – center for auditory and visual reflexes.

Pons – the bridge between two halves of the cerebellum.

Medulla Oblongata – communication and receiver center for motor fibers from the brain to the spinal cord and sensory fibers from the spinal cord to the brain.

Cerebellum (meaning "little brain") – responsible for balance and coordination and a wide range of functions and processes in the brain and body. It holds more than half of the neurons in the whole body. It is located at the bottom of the brain near the back of the head.

The Diencephalon is the structure that processes sensory and motor information and is very important in the autonomic control of muscles and organs. It regulates memory and emotion, coordinates motor movements, and works with the primary senses, such as hearing or seeing.

Thalamus – the information relay station for all memory, sensation (except smell), and pain impulses. It is responsible for processing all the information from the body's senses (except smell) before sending it to the cerebral cortex for interpretation. It is essential in sleep, wakefulness, consciousness, learning, and memory.

The hypothalamus is located deep in the brain and regulates the autonomic nervous system (fluid balance, temperature regulation, hormonal secretion, hunger, sleep, blood pressure, and emotions). Its primary function is to maintain the body in homeostasis and manage hormones. If damaged, many bodily functions will be affected.

Pituitary Gland – the master gland that controls hormone release from other glands:

1. Anti-diuretic hormone (ADH)
2. Adrenocorticotropic Hormone (ACTH)
3. Thyroid-stimulating hormone (TSH)
4. Follicle-stimulating hormone (FSH)
5. Growth Hormone (GH)
6. Melanocyte-stimulating hormone (MSH)

The reflex exam is fundamental to neurological examination. When motor neuron lesions are suspected, the reflex exam helps the clinician identify the location of the injury.

REFLEXES

Reflexes are involuntary responses or contractions of the muscles that occur when a stimulus is applied. Reflexes are classified as deep tendon, superficial, or pathological.

Most Common Reflexes Tested	
Biceps	Just anterior to the elbow
Triceps	Just posterior to the elbow
Brachioradialis	About 2-4 inches above the wrist on the radial aspect of the forearm
Quadriceps (Patella)	Just below the patella
Achilles (Ankle)	Just behind the ankle

Rating reflexes can be subjective. The force used to produce a response depends on the reflexes' response. Sometimes, clinicians prefer to indicate reflexes as "present, absent, or diminished" rather than using the grading scale.

Reflex Grading	
4+	Hyperactive with sustained *clonus* (involuntary rhythmic muscular spasms or contractions)
3+	Hyperactive

Hyperactive reflexes indicate that the lesion is a *CNS lesion*.

2+	Normal

Hypoactive or absent reflexes indicate that the lesion is a *PNS lesion.*

1+	Hypoactive
0	Absent

When the reflex seems to be diminished or absent, use *reinforcement*. Reinforcement is the contraction of other muscles to increase the reflex response assessed.

Reinforcement Used to Increase Reflex Activity or Response	
Arm Reflexes	Clench the teeth or squeeze both knees together.
Legs Reflexes	Lock fingers together and pull one hand against the other.

During the deep tendon reflexes assessment, *remember* to:

1. Joints should be at 90 degrees bend.
2. Check for asymmetry. Compare the reflexes on one side of the body to another (left and right).
3. Check for weakness or atrophy.
4. Use only enough force to produce a response.
5. Use reinforcement to increase the reflex response.

Upper Motor Neuron Defect (Above T6)	Lower Motor Neuron Defect (Below T6)
Spastic paralysis	Flaccid paralysis
No significant muscle atrophy	Significant muscle *atrophy* (muscle shrink)
Hyperreflexia	Hyporeflexia
+Babinski	-Babinski
Need to stimulate elimination.	Manual stool removal and straight catheterization

Cranial Nerves	
Nerve	Assessment
I - Olfactory	Smell
II - Optic	Visual Acuity (Snellen Chart)
III - Oculomotor	Pupils (PERLA), *Gaze*
IV - Trochlear	*Gaze* in all directions.
V - Trigeminal	Clench teeth and move jaw side-to-side.
VI - Abducens	*Gaze* in all directions.
VII - Facial	Smile, frown, raise eyebrows.
VIII - Auditory	Hear spoken word
IX - Glossopharyngeal	Gag reflex: Say “Ah” (observe palate and pharynx movement)
X - Vagus	Say “Ah” (observe palate and pharynx movement)

XI – Spinal Accessory	Shrug shoulders
XII - Hypoglossal	Stick tongue out, move it side to side, say “Ah” (observe palate and pharynx movement)

CHAPTER 10 THE MUSCULOSKELETAL SYSTEM

The musculoskeletal system is essential for movement, stability, shape, and support. It consists of two main parts: the muscular system, which includes all muscle types, and skeletal muscles that facilitate movement by acting on the joints.

DIAGNOSTIC TESTS

Laboratory Values

Sedimentation Rate (Sed Rate) – Erythrocyte Sedimentation Rate. This test is used to determine and monitor inflammation in the body. The normal value is males $\leq$ 15 mm/hour and females $\leq$ 2 mm/hour. It can be slightly elevated in elderly people. False positives can be shown in patients with *leukemia* or *polycythemia vera*.

Rheumatoid Factor - This test indicates rheumatoid arthritis. The normal value is 14 IU/ml.

Lupus Erythematosus Preparation (LE Prep)—This test determines if there are Lupus cells in the system. It is used in conjunction with the ANA test. If lupus cells were found in the LE Prep and the ANA test was negative, the patient was diagnosed with lupus. The LE Prep has been replaced for the ANA test discussed below. Its discontinuation is because "it is labor intensive, requires a special tube, and cannot be automated."

Antinuclear Antibodies (ANA) – The ANA test identifies antinuclear antibodies. These antibodies attack the person's tissue by directly attacking the cell's nucleus. This test is used when there is a suspicion of lupus, scleroderma, or rheumatoid arthritis.

Anti-dsDNA—The anti-dsDNA test is one of the first tests ordered when the doctor suspects the patient has an autoimmune disease or disorder, such as lupus.

C-Reactive Protein (CRP)—The liver makes this protein, which indicates an inflammatory process in the body.

Uric Acid—Uric acid is a waste product produced when the body breaks down purines. Purines are chemical compounds found in some food or drinks and can also be produced naturally by the body. Uric acid is filtered through the kidneys. If the kidneys are not functioning adequately, the accumulation of uric acid crystals in the joints will cause inflammation and pain, called Gout.

X-rays and Scans

Bone Scan – A bone scan utilizes nuclear imaging to help diagnose types of bone disease.

Arthroscopy—This is a minimally invasive surgical procedure in which a small tube with a fiber optic camera attached is inserted into a joint when there are joint problems.

Arthrocentesis—Also known as joint aspiration, this procedure treats bursitis, tendonitis, knee effusion, or septic arthritis.

Myelogram—This is an X-ray of the spinal canal. It involves a lumbar puncture. Contrast dye is injected, and the space in the spinal canal, nerve roots, and spinal cord can be visualized.

Electromyography (EMG) – This test helps diagnose and evaluate the function of the nerves and how they transmit to the skeletal muscles.

DISORDERS OF THE MUSCULOSKELETAL SYSTEM

FRACTURES

Types

Pathological – Fractures that happen because the bone is weak due to a disease such as osteoporosis.

Simple/Closed – The continuity of the bone cracks or breaks.

Compound – The bone breaks into tissue; bone shifts out of place. Requires OR.

Greenstick – Also known as a pediatric fracture or partial thickness fracture. It is called greenstick because it resembles the break of a green twig. One side of the bone is intact.

Comminuted – In this fracture, the bone is crushed and is critical. Crepitus (crunching noise) can be heard.

Spiral – These are signs of abuse and should be notified to the authorities.

FRACTURE TREATMENTS

When assessing fractures, follow the 5 "Ps": pain, Pallor, paresthesia (neuropathy), Paralysis, and *Pulselessness.*

Fractures are at risk of developing infection. Patients are also at *risk for clots (fat embolisms).* Monitor the patient for restlessness, which can be a sign of clots.

Fractures are cast for immobility. Cast care includes using an air dry or low-setting fan, pillows, neurovascular assessment, and monitoring for hot spots and odors.

Traction stabilizes a fracture or injury and helps restore tension to the surrounding tissues, muscles, and tendons.

Types

Skin Traction

Buck's—This is used to restore bone alignment and is used in physical therapy. It is beneficial for femur fractures. Straight pull on the extremity.

Russell's – Used to pull contracted muscles.

Bryant's – Vertical fraction used in infants with femur fractures.

Intermittent cervical/pelvic traction on top of clothes. Patients can remove the traction, but only the nurse can reapply it.

Skeletal Traction

Thomas/Pearson Attachment - Thomas Splint Pearson Attachments enhance lower leg support for patients with fractured femurs. They attach to the Thomas Splint at the knee and use a canvas or bandage sling for knee flexion. A footplate at the end supports the foot in a neutral position.

Halo - Halo-gravity traction is a technique for gradually correcting severe spinal deformities like scoliosis and kyphosis. Primarily used for children and adolescents, it can also help adults with significant spinal curvature.

Crutchfield Tongs—A traction device featuring pins inserted into the skull to distract and immobilize the neck. Crutchfield tongs are utilized to stabilize fractures of the cervical spine.

Nursing Care

Mobility will be impaired, and there is a potential for skin breakdown and infection. Nurses are responsible for positioning the patient using the weights and providing care to the ping site.

COMPLICATIONS OF FRACTURES

Fat Embolism Syndrome (FES)

This could happen within twelve hours after the injury and up to 72 hours after a major bone fracture. Major bones have more fat tissue, putting the patient at risk for developing FES.

Signs and Symptoms

The main sign is the development of *Adult Respiratory Distress Syndrome* (ARDS) with rapid breathing. Patients may develop a fever of >103. Other signs include pallor. If bleeding occurs under the skin, the patient will develop a petechia rash, usually visible on the chest, axillary, head, and neck. Confusion and lethargy are also common symptoms.

Treatment

Administration of O2, fluids, and steroids. Positive End-Expiratory Pressure (PEEP) is the positive pressure that remains in the lungs at the end of the respiratory cycle. This "pressure is greater than the atmospheric pressure in patients receiving mechanical ventilation" (Mora Carpio & Mora, 2022).

Compartment Syndrome

This complication is related to pressure from edema or bleeding that occurs during a fracture. It can also be related to casts or dressings applied too tight, which affect muscles, nerves, and blood vessels.

Signs and Symptoms

The patient will experience pain, paresthesia, and edema. Assess the 5 "Ps": Pain, Pallor, Pulseless, Paresthesia, and Pressure. Paresthesia is the first symptom.

Treatment

The physician will perform a surgical procedure known as *fasciotomy.* During a fasciotomy, the thin connective tissue or fascia that covers or separates the muscles and internal organs is removed to reduce pressure.

Ice can be applied, and the extremity will be elevated above the waist during the first twenty-four to forty-eight hours.

ASSISTIVE DEVICES FOR AMBULATION

Cane – Supports the uninvolved side.

Walker – The affected leg goes first.

Crutches – The crutches should be positioned two inches below the axilla, one inch below the axillary fold/line, and six inches from the foot.

For all the devices mentioned, the elbow should be at 30-degree flexion.

GAITS	USE
Swing thru	Lower extremities paralysis (paraplegia) with bracing
Swing to	Lower extremities paralysis (paraplegia) with bracing
Two-point gait (Similar to parallel Bars)	Assistive walking with the use of the crutch with the opposing leg
Three-point gait	Non-weight bearing (NWB). Two crutches and one good leg
Four-point gait	Lower extremities crippled, i.e., Spina Bifida.

DISORDERS OF THE HIP

Hip Fracture

Nursing Care

Patients will use Buck's Traction. The nurse will use the abductor splint or pillows between the legs for positioning. The patient will be centered in bed. Anti-embolic stockings will be applied, and the Sequential Compression Device (SCD) will provide active compression alternating from one lower extremity to the other. Range of Motion (ROM) will be provided to the unaffected extremity. During meals, the patient can be sitting in a semi-fowler position. The patient will be on anticoagulation medication.

Total Hip Replacement

This is a surgical replacement of the acetabulum and head of the femur (arthroplasty) with prosthesis. After surgery, the hip cannot be extended (abduction) more than 90 degrees because it can dislocate the extremity.

Nursing Care

The main goal is to prevent hip flexion contracture and infection. The nursing team will assess for signs and symptoms of bleeding, infection, contracture, constipation, or incontinence. Isometric exercises will be offered. Teaching for the patient and family should include using stairs precautions, promotion of sleep, dependent position for sex, and avoidance of bending, heavy lifting, jogging, and jumping. The patients will need prophylactic antibiotics before dental or dirty procedures and without driving for six weeks.

If the patient returns to the hospital with a possible infection, it puts the patient at risk for amputation. The patient will require antibiotics for approximately two years.

Osteomyelitis

Acute or chronic infection of the bone and surrounding tissues. The cause is usually a nosocomial (infection or disease developed in the hospital setting) infection such as *staph aureus*. It is diagnosed through a wound or incision culture. This condition is difficult to cure. The patient will be on long-term antibiotics.

On chronic osteomyelitis, the physician will perform a *sequestrectomy*. This is the removal of dead bone tissue.

Nursing Care

The affected area must be immobilized, and the patient should be placed in contact isolation with the health care providers, donning a gown and gloves. The patient will be on analgesics, and wound dressing changes will be sterile. Range of Motion (ROM) will be performed on unaffected extremities.

DISORDERS OF THE SPINE

Herniated Nucleus Pulposus (HNP)

In other words, a herniated vertebral disc. The test used to diagnose this is the myelogram. Treatments include traction, bed rest, anti-inflammatory medications (NSAIDS, Aleve), muscle relaxants, and heat and cold compresses. The surgeon can perform a *laminectomy* or laser discectomy.

Laminectomy

A laminectomy is an invasive surgical procedure used to remove small pieces of the lamina (back part of the vertebrae) or a spinal disc. The doctor may opt for a laser discectomy. There are two types of laminectomy procedures: Lumbar and Cervical.

Nursing Care

For lumbar laminectomies, the patients should be logrolled as long as they remain supine for at least the first twelve hours. They must remain flat. It is essential to assess the plantar dorsi/plantar. For cervical laminectomies, patients are kept in a low Fowler's position. The hand grasp and push strength must be evaluated. Another way to assess the hands is by asking the patients to wiggle their fingers. The patients need to ambulate to keep the calcium in the bones.

Spinal Fusion

For this procedure, the spinous processes are fused with bone grafts created from the patient's iliac crest or a donor.

Nursing Care

The nursing care will be the same as the one provided for laminectomy. The teaching includes encouraging activities such as ambulation. The patient should avoid prolonged sitting. The patients must be instructed to sit up at 90 degrees.

DISEASES OF THE MUSCULOSKELETAL SYSTEM

Osteoporosis

Osteoporosis is a condition that weakens bones, making them less dense. As people age, their bones lose their density and the ability to regrow. This starts to occur after 35 years old. Osteoporosis is more common in people over 50, especially women. Bone density is associated with estrogen levels. Risk factors include family history and people who consume alcohol and smoke. Some conditions associated with osteoporosis include endocrine disorders, gastrointestinal conditions, and blood disorders. The use of medications has been associated with the development of osteoporosis. This includes diuretics, hormone therapy, the use of steroids and antiacids, and blood thinners. A sedentary life can also lead to the development of osteoporosis.

Osteoporosis and Cancer

Cancer is a risk factor for osteoporosis. Elderly female patients are at risk for developing osteoporosis due to a decrease in estrogen levels in the system. Small-framed and non-obese Caucasians are also at risk. Increased amounts of coffee intake, smoking, and alcohol are risk factors. To prevent calcium loss, encourage the patient to exercise, mainly walking, because it will help the patient hold calcium in the bones.

Rheumatoid Arthritis (RA)

This is a chronic *autoimmune* disease ~~or condition~~ that causes inflammatory changes in joints and body systems. It is a systemic disease and the joints and systems are always stiff. Joints will be swollen and stiff for more than thirty minutes. The patients may experience fever, hypertension (HTN), and eye changes. Signs and symptoms will present symmetrically, and extremities will be red and hot. Patients who develop RA are at risk for renal failure.

Nursing Care

The goal is to prevent further joint destruction, relieve pain, and help reduce inflammation. Nursing care involves isometric exercises, and it is essential to provide pain medication before performing the exercises. Hot baths and ice packs help with signs and symptoms. Joints should remain in *extension* and not flexion.

One complication is the development of *bony ankylosis*, which is the union or fusion of the bones of a joint caused by the loss of cartilage. It results in complete immobility. Swimming, walking, and biking are encouraged.

Raynaud's Syndrome

In this condition, the small arteries narrow, reducing the amount or volume of blood that supplies the skin (*vasospasm*). The presentation of this condition is for fingers and toes to look pale and feel cold and numb. This condition can be treated, and these signs and symptoms should be reported to the physician immediately.

Arthritis Medications

ASA – Take this medication with food.

NSAIDS – Medications ending with "in, en, ene, il, ac." Examples: *Ibuprofen, Naproxen, Etodolac (Lodine), Diclofenac (Voltaren), Relafen, Meclomen, Oxaprozin, Indomethacin, Feldene, Clinoril.* These medications could cause aplastic anemia. Adverse reactions include rash, peripheral edema, fluid retention, tinnitus, and bronchospasm, and can affect the GI tract and the BP.

Laboratory tests include BUN, Creatinine, K, blood sugar, uric acid, and liver enzymes.

Nursing Care

Monitor the BP. The BUN, Creatinine, K, blood sugar, and liver enzymes should be monitored constantly. The K goes high. Encourage patients to use sunscreen. Give medications with food and avoid giving diuretics or antihypertensive medications at the same time.

COX 2 Inhibitors – These are anti-inflammatory medications. Celecoxib (Celebrex) is the only medication approved in the United States. It can cause heart attacks.

Steroids – The name of these medications ends with "lone, sone", for example, *Dexamethasone, Beclomethasone, Prednisone, Cortisone, Prednisolone, and Triamcinolone*. Patients on steroids should *avoid live vaccines*. Steroids are used under severe exacerbation. Adverse reactions include the development *of Cushing's Disease*.

Cushing's Disease

Cushing's disease develops if the person produces high levels of cortisol (hormone) or when a person is taking steroids for a prolonged time. Characteristics seen in people with Cushing's are a fatty hump between the shoulders, a rounded face, and pink or purple stretch marks on the body. Cushing causes cataracts with long-term use of steroid medications and affects the GI system. The patients will retain sodium, which causes edema and weight gain. Patients develop acne rash, insomnia, hypertension, and increased appetite. Laboratory tests include blood sugar (which will be increased), calcium, and K levels (which will be decreased).

Nursing Care

Monitoring electrolytes, BP, blood sugar, and daily weight is essential. Encourage a low-sodium diet and increase K intake. Education should include avoiding crowds and germs and weaning off steroid medication. Avoid giving steroids at the same time as giving Coumadin.

Disease Monitoring Anti-Rheumatic Drugs (DMARD)—These medications stop inflammation and decrease the body's ANA levels (Antinuclear Antibodies). Avoid live vaccines while taking these medications, such as Etanercept (which prevents the RA from progressing).

Methotrexate (MTX) is a drug used to treat various cancers, RA, MS, and Lupus (SLE). It should not be given on an empty stomach, and patients taking this medication should avoid consuming alcohol, NSAIDS, and DMARDs.

OSTEOARTHRITIS

This chronic non-systemic disease causes cartilage degeneration between the joints (DJD=Degenerative Joint Disease). It appears due to aging, obesity, or trauma. Signs and symptoms include joint pain, stiffness, and joint deformity. It is diagnosed through X-rays. Medications used include ASA or NSAIDS and steroid injections.

Nursing Care

The patient will have a limited range of motion (ROM). Nurses should alternate *Activities of Daily Living* (ADLs) to compensate for lack of mobility. Encourage patients to go for periods of walks or swim, but do not encourage bicycling. If a patient diagnosed with osteoarthritis complains of chest pain, the patient may have taken COX 2 in the past.

GOUT

Risk factors for the development of this condition include high intake of alcohol, a diet high in purine, starvation, heredity, renal failure, and Multiple Myeloma. Signs and symptoms include pain, redness, and swelling of the joint. This condition is diagnosed through laboratory tests such as uric acid level, which will be elevated in blood (>7mg/dL). The use of X-rays helps diagnose the condition.

Medications ordered to treat gout include Colchicine for acute gout, Probenecid, and Allopurinol for chronic gout. Colchicine is given until pain relief occurs. Probenecid dissolves urate deposits. For Allopurinol, it is essential to push fluids.

Nursing Care

Protect the feet using a cradle, promote rest, and use heat and cold therapy. Encourage a diet low in purine, proteins, and acids. Teaching should include reducing alcohol intake, shellfish, lentils, peas, beans, sweetbreads, mussels, organ meats, anchovies, mushrooms, spinach, and cauliflower.

Lupus Erythematosus (SLE)

This condition is chronic. Lupus is an autoimmune disease that destroys connective tissue involving multiple organ systems. It is fatal. African American women have a genetic disposition. Signs and symptoms include a butterfly-shaped rash on the cheeks and over the nose (facial erythema). Patients complain of fatigue, alopecia, oral mucosa, ulcerations photosensitivity, and Raynaud's disorder with decreased hand circulation related to vasospasms.

Several laboratory tests are ordered for patients with suspicion of having Lupus. The tests include ESR, Hgb, HCT, WBCs, PLTs, LE Prep, ANA, and VDRL. Venereal Disease Research Laboratory (VDRL) test will give a false positive. The treatment for patients with Lupus is non-specific and includes palliative care, steroids, NSAIDS, and plasmapheresis. Plasmapheresis is a process where plasma is separated from the blood cells. The plasma is then either replaced with a saline solution or albumin. Plasma can also be treated and then returned to the body. Lupus can be treated with different drugs that are usually used for cancer patients. These drugs include Cyclophosphamide or Methotrexate.

Nursing Care

Nursing care includes pain control and nutrition. Patients are encouraged to avoid the sun, hair dye, and spray, and the use of contraceptives and pregnancy. Stress can also exacerbate the condition and the symptoms.

AMPUTATION

Surgical removal of an extremity. The patient receives a visit from a rehabilitated amputee. Patients are encouraged to verbalize feelings and are educated in arm/hand exercises to build crutch strength. This is a massive alteration in body image, and the patient is at risk of infection.

Nursing Care

After surgery, it is essential to maintain the stump elevated for twenty-four hours only, which is then prone to prevent hip flexion contracture. The patient will experience what is known as "phantom limb sensation and pain." For this, the patient will not receive medication as the first intervention. The patient is instructed to tell the brain that the leg is gone. Guided imagery helps reduce feelings of anxiety and stress. Set a short-term goal with the patient. An example of a small goal is "being able to move from the bed to the commode or the chair."

CARPAL TUNNEL SYNDROME

Carpal tunnel syndrome is the compression of the median nerve caused by excessive wrist flexion. Signs and symptoms include palmar and wrist-to-shoulder pain. Patients also experience paresthesia, which can lead to paralysis. Treatment includes splints and surgery.

CONTINUOUS PASSIVE MOTION DEVICES (CPMD)

These devices help provide and maintain range of motion to a joint. They are usually prescribed after surgery. The devices assist with flexion and extension of the joint, usually the knee, without weight-bearing in knee arthroplasty patients. This equipment is integrated into therapy routines, enhancing the outcome of the postoperative recovery.

Benefits include accelerated recovery, reduced joint pain and stiffness, a lower incidence of thrombophlebitis, and improved blood circulation.

MYASTHENIA GRAVIS - Muscle Weakness

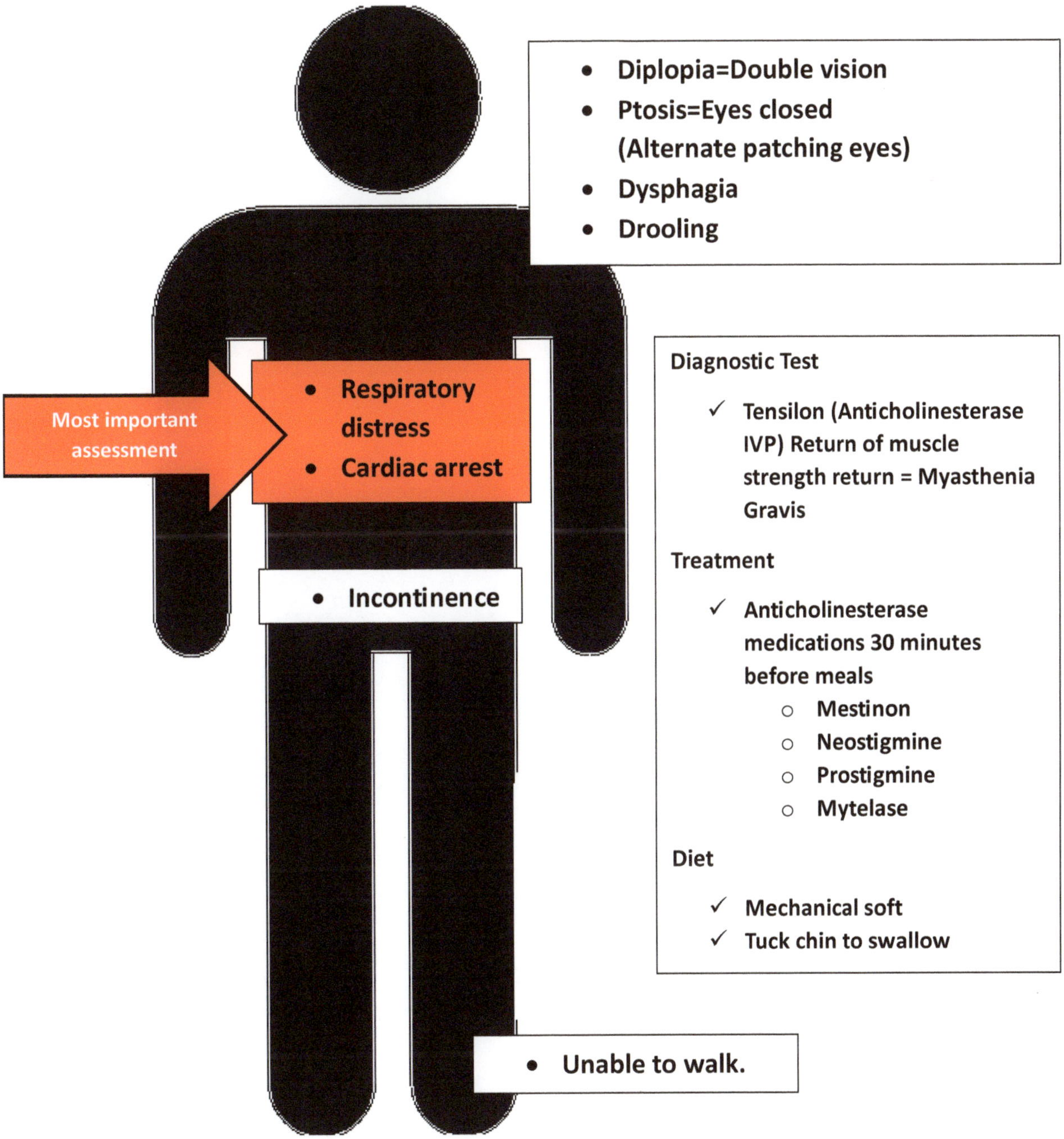

Diagnostic Test

- ✓ Tensilon (Anticholinesterase IVP) Return of muscle strength return = Myasthenia Gravis

Treatment

- ✓ Anticholinesterase medications 30 minutes before meals
    - Mestinon
    - Neostigmine
    - Prostigmine
    - Mytelase

Diet

- ✓ Mechanical soft
- ✓ Tuck chin to swallow

CHAPTER 11

THE IMMUNE AND LYMPHATIC SYSTEMS

The immune system, a powerful defender of the body against microorganisms, not only prevents illnesses but also aids in recovery from them. To strengthen it, increase the intake of nutritious foods, regular exercise, and sufficient sleep.

The lymphatic system, a complex network of organs, vessels, and tissues, protects against infections and plays a vital role in maintaining the body's fluid balance. Its critical organs, including bone marrow, thymus, and lymph nodes, are key to its functions. Swollen lymph nodes can indicate common infections like strep throat or more severe conditions such as cancer.

The IMMUNE SYSTEM is a complex combination of cells, organs, and tissues collaborating with all body systems. Its function is to protect the person from microorganism-causing diseases. When potent microorganisms interrupt homeostasis, it is difficult, if not impossible, for the immune system to protect the body system; the person is considered *immunocompromised*.

TYPES OF IMMUNITY

Innate or Nonspecific Immunity

This type of immunity protects the person from disease in general through three kinds of defenses we are born with: *anatomical defense* or barrier, *physiological defense* or barrier, and the *inflammatory response*.

Anatomical Defense

This defense includes the skin and mucous membranes, which help prevent bacteria, viruses, and other microorganisms from invading the body. Mucous secretions, saliva, and tears help protect the body by washing away substances that will compromise the immune system.

Physiological Defense

This type of defense includes body temperature and the acidity of specific organs. Microorganisms cannot tolerate high temperatures or high acidity. When the body identifies microorganisms, it increases the temperature by running a fever to signal that a foreign organism is threatening homeostasis. The stomach's acidity prevents bacteria from growing there.

When an organism invades an organ or tissue, the immune system sends disease-fighting cells and reinforcement to attack and protect the area. This action causes the area to become inflamed and swollen as an Inflammatory Response. This is another signal indicating that foreign organisms infect the organ or tissue.

Adaptive or Specific Immunity

When specific diseases attack the body, the body responds by making different types of cells or substances to fight those diseases.

Lymphocytes

Lymphocytes are specialized white cells. There are two kinds of lymphocytes: *B cells* and *T cells*. B cells produce antibodies to fight specific diseases. T cells destroy toxins and substances detrimental to the body's homeostasis.

Antigens

When the person is exposed to a specific disease, the foreign substance learns to create a response called *antigen* to fight back against the body's barriers or response. After being exposed to an antigen, the immune system, specifically the B cells, produces *antibodies* to fight the antigens the microorganisms create. The antibodies fit the antigen as a lock and key. The antibodies lock the antigen and destroy it. The antibodies continue in the plasma, preventing the disease from attacking the person again.

Acquired immunity is immunity a person gains actively or passively. *Active Immunity* is acquired through fighting the disease and creating antibodies or by receiving the vaccine against the disease. *Passive Immunity* is obtained when the baby is born, and the mother's antibodies (natural form) are passed on to the baby. Passive immunity can also be obtained through the intravenous administration of antibodies from someone who was infected before with the same disease.

THE LYMPHATIC SYSTEM

The LYMPHATIC SYSTEM removes excess fluids and waste products found in the tissues that disrupt homeostasis at the cell level. The lymphatic system helps fight infections and works closely with the immune and circulatory systems. This system comprises lymphoid organs, lymph nodes, vessels, and capillaries. The fluid that circulates throughout the structures is called *lymph*. Unlike the pumped blood, the lymphatic system has valves preventing the unfiltered lymph from backing up. This transparent yellow fluid carries the lymphocytes discussed in the previous section. When foreign microorganisms enter the body, the lymph nodes become enlarged or swollen. This is another alarm the body uses to indicate that the body is fighting an infection. After the lymph is filtered and microorganisms and waste products are removed, the lymph returns to the bloodstream. The lymph nodes are located throughout the body: the neck, armpit, chest, abdomen, extremities, and groin.

CONDITIONS

Human Immunodeficiency Virus (HIV)

There are two types of HIV: HIV-1 and HIV-2. HIV-2 is not highly transmissible. Research is still being conducted regarding this type. HIV-1 is severe and highly transmissible. The modes of transmission are blood, mucus, intercourse (anal and vaginal sex), and breast milk. The human immunodeficiency virus destroys the T cells, specifically the CD4. The CD4/T cells are the cells that fight microorganisms. There are four groups that HIV-1 can be broken into M, N, O, and P. HIV occurs in stages.

Stage 1 – Acute HIV Infection

During this stage, the person is highly contagious and may not know they are infected. After the person has been infected, and within two to four weeks after the infection, the person will develop flu-like symptoms.

Stage 2 – Clinical Latency (HIV Inactivity)

This stage can last ten years or more. The virus is active but not reproducing at high levels. The person will not experience symptoms of infection. If the person is on antiretroviral therapy, this stage can last several decades. Towards the end of this stage, the virus starts to multiply rapidly. At the same time, the CD4 count decreases. At that time, the person begins to have more signs and symptoms.

Stage 3 – Acquired Immunodeficiency Syndrome (AIDS)

When the CD4 cell count drops below 200 cells/mm, the person is diagnosed with this disease. The virus has damaged the immune system, and evidence of the signs and symptoms will increase. Symptoms of this stage are chills, fever, sweating, swollen lymph nodes and glands, weakness, and weight loss. During the last stage of the disease, the patient will develop what is called *AIDS Dementia Complex*.

HIV spreads to the brain, developing encephalopathy, an infection that affects the brain, resulting in the AIDS Dementia Complex. The greater the infection, the worse the dementia symptoms. The person will experience swelling brain membranes and spinal column, memory loss, cognitive impairment, difficulty concentrating and speaking, apathy, and reduced coordination of motor skills.

DIAGNOSTIC TESTS

Nucleic Acid Test (NAT): This expensive but accurate-can identify HIV in its early stages.

Antigen/Antibody Test: This test looks for the antibodies and antigens in the blood, finding them within two to six weeks of infection.

Antibody Test: The most common antibody tests are the *ELISA (EIA)* and *Western Blot* tests performed on oral fluid.

Treatment

Antiretroviral Therapy reduces the virus in the blood and the body fluids. This therapy has been critical in the management of HIV, providing better care and a better quality of life to immunocompromised patients with HIV. If the virus is not managed on time or appropriately, it will eventually destroy the immune system without hope of being rehabilitated.

CHAPTER 12 GERONTOLOGICAL NURSING

According to the World Health Organization (2022), by 2050, the proportion of older adults over 60 will double from 12% to 22%. The United Nations Vision for 2050 promotes the development of a healthcare infrastructure that meets those needs. This chapter covers normal changes in aging, conditions that affect mainly older adults, ways to assess older adults, negligence and abuse, and the importance of increased knowledge in dementia.

CHANGES OF NORMAL AGING

I. Neurologic
  a. Decreased
    i. Number and size of brain cells
    ii. Amount of neurotransmitters
  b. Increased reaction time (Taking longer to formulate thoughts)
  c. Nursing Implications
    i. Assess sleep, memory, response, and reaction time.
    ii. Nursing diagnosis
      1. Alteration of thought processes
      2. Alteration of sleep patterns
    iii. Nursing Interventions
      1. Provide more time to perform tasks.
      2. Provide more time to answer/respond.
      3. Maintain nighttime routines.
      4. Promote daily orientation with calendars, clocks, and visits.

II. Neurosensory
  a. Hearing
    *i. Presbycusis (*Progressive hearing loss)
      1. High frequency tones are lost first (Decreased acuity to high pitch sounds)
      2. Sounds may be distorted (May have difficulty understanding words when there is background noise)
  b. Vision
    i. The lens becomes opaque.
    ii. Decreased visual field.

iii. Decreased color discrimination.

iv. Presbyopia (farsightedness due to decreased accommodation)

v. Pupillary changes with loss of light responsiveness.

Difficulty adapting to darkness. Difficulty seeing in dim light.

c. Taste

i. Number of taste buds

ii. Dulled taste sensation. Especially for bitter, sour, or salty flavors.

d. Smell (Olfactory)

i. Olfactory sense decreases

e. Touch (Tactile)

i. Sense of touch dulled.

ii. Pain threshold higher

iii. The sense of vibration decreased.

f. Vestibular/Kinesthetic changes

i. Decreased proprioception.

ii. Decreased coordination.

iii. Decreased equilibrium.

g. Nursing implications

i. Assess normal physiological changes.

h. Nursing Diagnosis

i. Alteration in sensory perception (specify)

ii. Potential to injury

iii. Impaired verbal communication

iv. Potential social isolation

v. Fear

vi. Anticipatory grieving

i. Nursing interventions

i. Lower tone of voice when speaking

ii. Reduce background noise before speaking.
iii. Determine if a patient uses hearing aids and if it is working.
iv. Determine if the patient uses eyeglasses/lenses.
v. Provide increased lighting.
vi. Provide night lights.
vii. Provide handrails.
viii. Promote expression of feelings.
ix. Provide touch.

III. Respiratory

a. Decreased
   i. Respiratory muscle tone
   ii. Functional alveoli
   iii. Ciliary action
   iv. Force of cough
   v. PO2
   vi. Response to increased O2 demand
b. Nursing diagnoses
   i. Ineffective airway clearance
   ii. Alteration in breathing patterns
   iii. Impaired gas exchange
   iv. Activity intolerance
c. Nursing interventions
   i. Assess respiratory problems.
   ii. Teach relaxation exercises, deep breathing, correct position, taking adequate liquids, and smoking cessation.
   iii. Encourage patient to take preventive vaccines (influenza and pneumococcal)
   iv. Provide rest periods.

IV. Cardiovascular

a. Decreased

i. Elasticity of heart and arteries.

ii. Increased systolic pressure (widening)

iii. Efficiency of heart and peripheral valves.

iv. Maximum heart rate with exercise.

b. Increased

i. Recovery time with exercise

ii. Peripheral resistance

iii. Formation of atherosclerotic plaques

c. Nursing implications

i. Assess CV functioning.

d. Nursing Diagnosis

i. Alteration in tissue perfusion is related to the interruption of arterial and venous flow.

ii. Activity intolerance.

iii. Fatigue

e. Nursing interventions

i. Provide for rest periods.

ii. Teach patients about following a low-salt diet and having regular health checkups, including blood pressure checks.

iii. Monitor for orthostatic hypertension.

Instruct the patient to move slowly when changing positions.

V. Musculoskeletal

a. Decreased

i. Height

ii. Muscle mass, tone, and strength.

If muscle is replaced by fat, the patient will lose strength.

b. Increased
    i. Joint and cartilage erosion
    ii. Thinning of vertebral
c. Nursing implications
    i. Assess strength and ability to walk.
d. Nursing diagnosis
    i. Impaired physical mobility
    ii. High risk for injury
e. Nursing interventions
    i. Teach the need to exercise.
    ii. Environmental safety
    iii. Need for calcium intake.

VI. Gastrointestinal
a. Decreased
    i. Esophageal peristalsis
    ii. External sphincter reflexes
    iii. Saliva production
    iv. Liver size, weight, and efficiency.
    v. Gastric acid secretion
    vi. Intestinal mobility
    vii. Metabolic and caloric needs
b. Nursing implications
    i. Assess swallowing, weight, and bowel function.
c. Nursing diagnoses
    i. Alteration in nutrition less than body requirements
    ii. Impaired swallowing
    iii. Alteration in elimination
        1. Constipation

2. Incontinence

d. Nursing interventions

i. Teach

1. Reduce caloric intake. This is accomplished by decreasing the fat and simple carbohydrates if we are overweight.
2. Maintain an amount of protein in the diet.
3. Need for adequate calcium, iron, and vitamins.
4. Need for increased fluids, fiber, roughage, and exercise.
5. Use of thickened fluids if impaired swallowing.

VII. Genitourinary

a. Decreased

i. Glomerular filtration rate
ii. Renal blood flow, mass, and nephrons
iii. Bladder muscle tone
iv. Sphincter tone
v. Vaginal secretions
vi. Size of testes
vii. Speed and force of ejaculation

b. Nursing implications

i. Assess urinary output and continence, vaginal itching and discomfort during intercourse, and sexual functioning.

c. Nursing diagnoses

i. Incontinence: stress, urge, overflow, functional
ii. Alterations in sexual patterns
iii. Knowledge deficit related to normal physical changes related to aging.

d. Nursing interventions

i. Encourage 2000 to 3000cc of fluids daily.

ii. Assess drug toxicity.

iii. Provide toileting and elimination needs.

iv. Administer diuretics by 4 pm

v. Teach Kegel exercises for incontinence.

vi. Provide privacy for intimacy.

VIII. Integumentary

a. Decrease

i. Circulation, number of cells, and elastic collagen fibers

ii. Pressure and light–touch sensation

iii. Production of sweat, sebum, and vitamin D

iv. Cell replacement results in thinning skin.

v. Hair color and amount

b. Increased

i. Itching of skin

ii. Dryness of skin

iii. Wrinkling

iv. Uneven pigmentation

v. Age spots and skin tags

vi. Occurrence of skin lesions

c. Nursing implications

i. Assess skin condition and discomfort.

d. Nursing diagnoses

i. Knowledge deficit: Normal changes and related skincare

ii. Potential alteration in skin integrity

iii. Body image disturbance

iv. Self-esteem disturbance

v. Alteration in oral mucus membrane

e. Nursing intervention

    i. Teach monitoring of skin condition, skin care, cleansing, and protection from sun.
    ii. Check skin turgor over sternum.
    iii. Facilitate expression of feelings regarding changes in appearance
    iv. Handle gently to prevent skin tears.

IX. Endocrine: Regulation, Temperature, and Infection

a. Decreased

    i. Secretion of growth hormone
    ii. Gonadal function with female menopause
    iii. Thyroid hormone production
    iv. Glucose tolerance
    v. Shivering
    vi. Functioning sweat glands
    vii. Temperature elevation response to infections
    viii. Tolerance to cold

b. Nursing implications

    i. Assess for activity tolerance and signs of infection other than temperature elevation.

c. Nursing diagnoses

    i. Fatigue/activity tolerance
    ii. Potential hypothermia related to exposure to a cold environment.
    iii. Hyperthermia is related to exposure to extreme temperatures.
    iv. Teach appropriate care during hot or cold weather.
    v. Monitor temperature and observe for signs and symptoms of infection.
    vi. Provide rest periods.

X. Cells

a. Decreased

i. Size

ii. Intracellular fluid

b. Nursing implications

The elderly are more susceptible to fluid balance problems.

MEDICATION PROBLEMS

I. Multiple medications – Rx and OTC

a. Danger of drug interaction

b. Assess drug toxicity and side effects.

II. Decreased liver and kidney function.

a. Half-life may be increased.

b. Danger of overdose

III. Self-Administration

a. May have difficulty taking the right drug at the right dose at the right time.

i. Check compliance with the amount of medication and time.

b. Color coding will be used to facilitate proper administration if necessary.

c. Determine if the patient can open the container.

d. Oral medications

i. Check swallowing.

ii. If swallowing difficulties appear:

1. Suggest liquid medication preparation if the patient is unable to swallow pills or capsules.
2. Crush large, non-enteric coated tablets.
3. Give a drink of water before medication to assure moist mucous membranes.
4. Give medication with pudding, applesauce, or ice cream.

e. Parenteral medications

i. Do not use immobile limbs.

1. Closely monitor the IV rate to avoid overhydration and the onset of pulmonary edema.

ELDER ABUSE

I. Definitions

a. Abuse

Willful, active actions briefly result in physical, psychosocial, and material harm.

b. Neglect

Failure to meet physical, psychosocial, or material needs.

II. Incidence of abuse occurs in homes and long-term and acute care institutions.

III. Characteristics of abused persons

a. Female more than male

b. Caucasians are more frequently abused.

c. Physical and/or cognitive impairments that make the patient dependent on others for ADL.

d. Display dependency characteristics

e. Exhibit problematic behavior.

i. Bossy, demanding.

ii. Incontinent

iii. Wandering

iv. Nighttime shouting

IV. Characteristics of the abuser

a. Is ill-prepared or reluctant to provide care.

b. Have unrealistic expectations of older people.

c. Lack of knowledge/skills required to provide care.

d. Have ineffective coping patterns.

e. Personal life in disarray

i. Problems with own children

ii. Marital conflict

iii. Personal physical/emotional problems

iv. Alcohol or drug abuse

v. Lack of communications skills.

1. Difficulty in verbally relating and sharing feelings.

f. Absence of support system.

V. Nursing Implications

a. Need for self-awareness.

i. Evaluate personal feelings towards own aging and towards older people.

ii. Become aware of personal attitude toward neglect/abuse.

iii. Acknowledge that every person is capable of being an abuser.

b. Assess for potential/active abuse.

i. Does a patient have high-risk characteristics?

ii. Does the caregiver have high-risk characteristics?

iii. Signs of abuse

1. Frequent visits to ED.

2. Multiple bruising, fractures, lacerations, and abrasions in various stages of healing

3. Evidence of burns, rope burns.

4. Head injury due to hair pulling.

5. Appear overmedicated.

6. Behavioral

a. Wariness of contact with adult

b. Very aggressive infantile behavior

c. Withdrawn

d. Expressing ambivalent feelings toward caregivers

iv. Signs of Neglect

1. Dehydration
2. Malnourishment
3. Poor hygiene
4. Inappropriate clothing

VI. Nursing Diagnoses

a. Potential for violence
b. Ineffective individual coping
c. Ineffective family coping: compromised/disabling.
d. Coping – potential for growth
e. Hopelessness
f. Knowledge deficit
g. Spiritual distress – guilt
h. Disturbance in self-concept – self-esteem
i. Potential for injury
j. Social isolation
k. Alteration in nutrition
l. Fluid balance deficit

VII. Nursing interventions

a. Promote safety.
    i. Report to the appropriate supervisor/social agency
    ii. Determine if a person needs to be removed.
b. Develop *IPR (Intellectual Property Rights*) with abuse.
c. Promote trust with consistency and care.
d. Promote self-esteem by providing affection and caring.
e. Ensure that basic needs are met.
f. Promote expression of feelings.
g. Communicate empathy with the abuser.
h. Explore resources available to abusers.

i. Refer to community resources.

    i. Daycare

    ii. Respite care

    iii. Self-help groups

    iv. Counseling servicer

j. Teach the abuser realistic expectations for the abused and how to provide care.

k. Document findings, interventions, evaluations

ASSESSMENT TOOL

Dr. Terry Fulmer, president of The John A. Hayford Foundation, developed the *Fulmer SPICES,* an assessment tool designed to identify health-related conditions associated with normal aging in older adults. The acronym SPICES helps to remember the problems associated with normal aging changes in the hospital setting. When assessing the older adult, the nurse should ask specific questions as indicated below.

Fulmer SPICES ASSESSMENT TOOL		
SPICES	EVIDENCE	
	Yes	No
Sleep Disorders • Ask about sleep and observe sleep patterns.		
Problems with Eating or Feeding • Evaluate appetite and food preferences and the ability to feed yourself.		
Incontinence • Observe voiding and bowel patterns and evaluate for causes of incontinence.		
Confusion • Establish baseline cognitive status and monitor for cognitive changes.		
Evidence of Falls		

• Ask about a history of falls and evaluate for additional risk factors.		
Skin Breakdown • Identify any skin breakdown and evaluate risk factors for skin breakdown.		

DEMENTIA AND THE OLDER ADULT

Dementia is medical terminology for symptoms affecting memory, thinking, and social skills. Dementia is not a normal part of aging, and the symptoms interfere with daily living activities. Memory loss is usually one of the first symptoms the person experiences concerning this condition. However, memory loss alone does not mean that the person has dementia. Signs and symptoms vary and include cognitive and psychological changes. The leading cause of dementia is *Alzheimer's Disease*.

Alzheimer's Disease

This condition develops through abnormalities created in the brain by depositing insoluble proteins called amyloid plaques. These plaques are not soluble and attach themselves to brain structures, causing damage to the neurons and other brain tissues. This condition starts slowly. Cognitive and psychosocial skills will be affected depending on the location in the amyloid plaques' brain. As the condition progresses, the person cannot identify family members. Patients also need help communicating and having trouble speaking, reading, and writing. Their behavior is altered, and they become aggressive and anxious. A person with this condition can live for decades. This condition is extremely taxing for the caregiver.

Nursing Care

The care offered to patients suffering from dementia should be age-friendly. Age-friendly care recognizes evidence-based interventions for older adults. These interventions address medication, mentation, mobility, and what the older adult considers essential in their life. Provide patient-centered care. This is important because it identifies older adults' care preferences and goals. Medication administration should be addressed while considering the patient's mentation mobility and preferences. Consider the following guidelines when offering care to a dementia patient:

- Do not rush the older adult during daily activities.
- Be patient
- Do not talk to the older adult as a child
- Provide dignified care
- Promote independence and self-care
- Divide tasks into simple steps
- Be mindful of body language and what message is being sent to the patient
- Demonstrate compassionate, caring, and empathetic behavior while interacting with the older adult
- Increase the knowledge and understanding of dementia
- Understand the caregiver's struggles and fatigue
- Educate the caregiver on how to handle the patient's care

Nurses and other clinical personnel, including caregivers caring for patients whose cognitive and psychosocial skills are declining, should receive training tailored to address dementia patient's unique issues.

Dementia Aware Competency Evaluation (D.A.C.E.)

The Dementia Aware Competency Evaluation (D.A.C.E.) is a crucial method designed by P.K. Beville, the founder of Second Wind Dreams. It assesses the competency of clinical personnel and their ability to be involved in caring for patients displaying signs and symptoms of dementia. The D.A.C.E. focuses on the caregiver's competency and observable areas such as sensitivity, empathy, and respect, emphasizing its importance in professional development.

Falls

Older adults are at an increased risk for falls. As people age, their reflexes and responses diminish, making it difficult for them to stop falling. They also experience increased difficulty understanding situations or making proper decisions.

Nursing Care

When providing nursing care to dementia patients, being patient and understanding is crucial. The nurse must assess the patient's history of falls, usually with the family's assistance. Observing the patient's behavior and body language is key to evaluating their confidence when standing or walking. The patient may feel anxious or unsteady. Be patient and reassure the patient using a calm voice. Knowing the patient's medications that may contribute to falls is also important. Before ambulation, ensure the patient wears eyeglasses if needed, proper shoes, and gets a set of orthostatic vital signs. A change in the systolic blood pressure above 20 mm Hg or diastolic blood pressure above 10 mm Hg increases the patient's risk of falling. The patient may feel lightheaded or dizzy when standing. It's important not to rush the patient through activities of daily living. Allow the patient to rest and breathe, demonstrating patience and understanding in your care.

Skin Assessment

A normal change of aging concerning the skin is a decrease in body mass and muscle waste, and the skin becomes thinner and fragile. Older adults' skin is easier to break. Wounds can be categorized as superficial wounds and deep wounds.

Nursing Care

Skin assessment must be performed daily. When assessing Superficial wounds, assess for wounds that do not heal, are draining, are red and swollen, have a foul smell, or you can observe debris inside the wound. Deep wounds must be assessed when the nurse observes the wound growing and not healing; when there is high temperature around the wound, the area is swollen or edematous, smells or new wounds can develop near the wound, or exposed bones can be seen. When performed on time, this assessment will decrease the risk of infection development.

WOUND ASSESSMENT			
SUPERFICIAL WOUNDS	DEEP WOUND	Yes	No
Non-healing wound	Size is bigger		
Exudative wound	Temperature increased		
Red and bleeding wound	Osteo (probe to exposed bone)		
Debris in the wound	New or satellite areas of breakdown		
Smell from the wound	Exudate, erythema, edema		
	Smell from the wound		

Sepsis and the Older Adult

Untreated wounds become reservoirs for bacteria and other pathogens, which can multiply and infect other body areas. The immune system sends cells specialized in regulating the inflammatory process in the body. These cells are called cytokines. Cytokines are trained to fight and destroy pathogens. If the wounds remain untreated, they can invade the circulatory system, reaching every area of the body. This increases cytokines, leading to an increased response in the inflammatory process, and resulting in organ damage. That is sepsis.

The older adult is at an increased risk for developing sepsis and experiencing a delayed response in treatment. As the person ages, they will experience a decrease in autoimmunity. Co-morbidities, chronic illnesses, and recurrent or long hospitalizations put the older adult at an increased risk for developing sepsis. Treatment is often delayed because signs and symptoms of sepsis may be missed. After all, older adults do not present infection in the same way as younger patients. In older adults, sepsis will present different symptoms like weakness, anorexia, malaise, falls, and urinary incontinence. Regardless of age being a risk factor, older adults respond well to timely and appropriate interventions.

Nursing Care

The nurse performs a complete head-to-toe assessment to identify signs and symptoms of infection. Prompt recognition of the source of infection should be communicated to the primary physician for immediate identification of treatment and its initiation. Blood tests will be conducted to identify electrolyte imbalances, abnormal liver or kidney function, and blood clotting issues. Treatment includes antibiotics, support therapy like oxygen or dialysis, IV fluids to balance out the electrolytes, and medication to increase the blood pressure. Education and emotional support for the patient and the family are very important.

RESOURCES

American Diabetes Association. (2024). *Prevention or Delay of Diabetes and Associated Comorbidities: Standards of Care in Diabetes.* 47 (Supplement_1): S43–S51. from https://doi.org/10.2337/dc24-S003

American Heart Association. (2024). *Cardiomyopathy.* https://www.heart.org/en/health-topics/cardiomyopathy

American Heart Association. (2022). Get with the guidelines-stroke. https://www.heart.org/en/professional/quality-improvement/get-with-the-guidelines/get-with-the-guidelines-stroke/recognition-from-get-with-the-guidelines-stroke

American Heart Association. (2022). Understanding Blood Pressure Readings. https://www.heart.org/en/health-topics/high-blood-pressure/understanding-blood-pressure-readings.

American Heart Association. (2015). *Transesophageal Echocardiogram*. https://www.heart.org/en/health-topics/heart-attack/diagnosing-a-heart-attack/transesophageal-echocardiography-tee.

Appel G. B. (1990). *Aminoglycoside nephrotoxicity.* The American journal of medicine, 88(3C), 16S–42S. https://doi.org/10.1016/0002-9343(90)90082-o

Armata, N.N. (2023). *Chvostek Sign*. https://www.osmosis.org/answers/chvostek-sign#How%20Is%20The%20Chvostek%20Sign%20Performed?

Bar-On, R. and Parker, J.D.A. (2000). The Handbook of Emotional Intelligence. Jossey-Bass Publishers. San Francisco, California.

Barrell, A. (2018). *What causes Bence Jones protein in urine?* https://www.medicalnewstoday.com/articles/321192#how-is-it-done

Bhandari, S. (2023). *What is a Uric Acid Test?* https://www.webmd.com/arthritis/uric-acid-blood-test

Brennan, D. (2021). *What is fetor hepaticus?* https://www.webmd.com/a-to-z-guides/what-is-fetor-hepaticus

Brennan, D. (2021). *What is Urine Specific Gravity?* https://www.webmd.com/a- to-z-guides/what-is-urine-specific-gravity

Britannica, T. Editors of Encyclopedia (2018). How are radioactive isotopes used in medicine? Encyclopedia Britannica. https://www.britannica.com/question/How-Buttner, R. and Burns, E. (2012). *Hypokalaemia.* https://litfl.com/hypokalaemia- ecg-library/are-radioactive-isotopes-used-in-medicine.

Centers for Disease Control and Prevention. (2017). *Stopping elderly accidents, deaths, & injuries (STEADI) Initiative*. www.cdc.gov/steadi/

Centers for Disease Prevention and Control. (2022). *LDL and HDL Cholesterol and Triglycerides.* https://www.cdc.gov/cholesterol/ldl_hdl.htm.

Centers for Disease Control and Prevention. (2018). *Common Reproductive Health Concerns for Women.* https://www.cdc.gov/reproductivehealth/womensrh/healthconcerns.html

Center for Disease Prevention and Control. (https://www.cdc.gov/sepsis/index.html

Christiano, D. (2018). *All About Fat Embolism Syndrome.* https://www.healthline.com/health/fat-embolism-syndrome#symptoms

Christiano, D. and Santos-Longhurst, A. (2021). *What causes asterixis, and how is it treated?* https://www.healthline.com/health/asterixis

Dementia Society. (2024). Dementia definitions. https://www.dementiasociety.org/definitions

Dementia Society. (2024). Dementia-like conditions.
https://www.dementiasociety.org/dementia-like-conditions

Dirkes, S.A., (2015). Acute kidney injury: Causes, phases, and early detection.
https://www.myamericannurse.com/acute-kidney-injury/?

End Sepsis Organization. (2024). Sepsis and the elderly. https://www.endsepsis.org/what-is-sepsis/sepsis-and-aging/

Frankenburg, W. K., & Dodds, J. B. (1967). The Denver Developmental Screening Test. The Journal of Pediatrics, 71(2), 181–191. https://doi.org/10.1016/S0022-3476(67)80070-2

Fernández-de Thomas, R.J., Munakomi, S., and De Jesús, O. (2023). *Craniotomy.*
https://www.ncbi.nlm.nih.gov/books/NBK560922/#:~:text=For%20surgery%20in%20the%20supratentorial, skull%20below%20the%20transverse%20sinus.

Fresenius. (2022). Hemodialysis Access: your lifeline for treatment.
https://www.freseniuskidneycare.com/treatment/in-center-hemodialysis/hemodialysis-access-options

Fulmer, T. (1991). *The Geriatric Nurse Specialist Role: A New Model.* Nursing Management, 22(3), 91- 93. https://niche.kdp.io/course/433/player/1210

Grabinski, C.J. (2007). *Gerontological nursing.* https://www.sciencedirect.com/

Heitz, D. (2018). *Plasmapheresis: What to Expect.*
https://www.healthline.com/health/plasmapheresis

Hertz, Y. (2018). *Potassium Imbalances in the ECG Illustration.*
https://www.pinterest.com/pin/454863631101269362/

Hewitt, N., Bucknall, T., & Faraone, N. M. (2016). Lateral positioning for critically ill adult patients. The Cochrane database of systematic reviews, 2016(5), CD007205. https://doi.org/10.1002/14651858.CD007205.pub2

Jain, S and Lindsay M. Iverson, LM. (2022). *Glasgow Coma Scale.* https://www.ncbi.nlm.nih.gov/books/NBK513298/

Kampfrath, T. (2023) *Anti-dsDNA Test.* https://www.testing.com/tests/anti-dsdna/

Khaku, A.S. and Tadi, P. (2022). *Cerebrovascular Disease.* https://www.ncbi.nlm.nih.gov/books/NBK430927/.

Khan, Z. (2023). *Cryoprecipitates.* https://www.medicinenet.com/cryoprecipitate/article.htm

Khatri, M. (2021). *Ulcerative colitis.* https://www.webmd.com/ibd-crohns-disease/ulcerative-colitis/what-is-ulcerative-colitis

Leonard, J., Whiteman, K., Stephens, K., Henry, C., and Swanson-Biearmann, B. (2022). Improving communication and collaboration skills in graduate nurses: An evidence-based approach. https://www.doi.org/10.3912/OJIN.Vol27No02Man03

Marcin, J. (2017). *Urine Osmolality Test.* https://www.healthline.com/health/osmolality-urine.

McCarthy, C. J., Behravesh, S., Naidu, S. G., & Oklu, R. (2016). Air Embolism: Practical Tips for Prevention and Treatment. Journal of clinical medicine, 5(11), 93. https://doi.org/10.3390/jcm5110093

McMillan, M.G. (2018). *How to do the right thing even when no one is watching.* "Ethical behavior is doing the right thing when no one else is watching—even when doing the wrong thing is legal."

Mealtime Partners, Inc. (2018). *Chin Positioning During Swallowing.* https://mealtimepartners.com/dining/chin_positioning_during_swallowing.htm

Medline Plus. (2023). *Caloric stimulation.* https://medlineplus.gov/ency/article/003429.htm#:~:text=How%20the%20Test%20is%20Performed&text=This%20test%20stimulates%20your%20acoustic, side%20eye%20movements%20called%20nystagmus.

Medline Plus. (2023). *Laboratory Tests.* https://medlineplus.gov/lab-tests.

Medscape. (2023). *Desmopressin.* https://reference.medscape.com/drug/ddavp-stimate-noctiva-desmopressin-342819.

Merriam-Webster Dictionary. (2024). Nurse. https://www.merriam-webster.com/dictionary/nurse

Mora-Carpio, A. and Mora, J. (2022). *Positive End-Expiratory Pressure.* https://www.ncbi.nlm.nih.gov/books/NBK441904/

Naderi-pour, A. (2015). *Specific Types of Traction.* https://www.orthopaedicsone.com/display/Review/Specific+Types+of+Traction

Nasa, P, Juneja, D. and Sinhg, O. (2012). Severe sepsis and septic shock in the elderly: overview. https://pmc.ncbi.nlm.nih.gov/articles/PMC3956061/

National Cancer Institute. (2023). *Adenoma.* https://www.cancer.gov/publications/dictionaries/cancer-terms/def/adenoma.

National Cancer Institute. (2024). Cancer treatment. https://www.cancer.gov/about-cancer/treatment/types/surgery

National Cancer Institute. (2024). Comprehensive cancer information. https://www.cancer.gov/

National Cancer Institute. (2023). *Reproductive system.* https://www.cancer.gov/publications/dictionaries/cancer-terms/def/reproductive-system

National Institute of Aging. (2022). *What is dementia? Symptom, Types, and diagnosis.* https://www.nia.nih.gov/health/alzheimers-and-dementia/what- dementia-symptoms-types-and-diagnosis

National Institute of Health. (2022). *Alkaline Phosphatase.* https://medlineplus.gov/lab-tests/alkaline-phosphatase/

National Institute of Health. (2022). *Hepatitis*. https://medlineplus.gov/lab-tests/hepatitis-panel/

Newman, G. (2020). *How to assess reflexes.* https://www.merckmanuals.com/professional/neurologic-disorders/neurologic-examination/how-to-assess-reflexes

Pagan, C.N. (2022). *Penile cancer.* https://www.webmd.com/cancer/penile-cancer-overview

Prescribers' Digital Reference. (2023). *SSKI.* https://www.pdr.net/drug-summary/SSKI-potassium-iodide-2783.

Rajkumar, V. and Waseem, M. (2022). Aldosteronism. https://www.ncbi.nlm.nih.gov/books/NBK555992/.

Roland, R. (2022). *Intussusception in Adults and Children.* https://www.healthline.com/health/intussusception#symptoms

Romanos-Sirakis EC, Desai D. (2023) ABO Blood Group System. StatPearls Publishing. https://www.ncbi.nlm.nih.gov/books/NBK580518/

Sarin, A. (2024). Common types of ostomies: Colostomy, Ileostomy, and Urostomy. https://health.ucdavis.edu/surgery/specialties/colorectal/ostomy/types.html

Second Wind Dreams. (2024) Dementia aware competency evaluation. https://secondwind.org/programs/dace/

Sibbald, R. G., Woo, K., & Ayello, E. A. (2006). *Increased bacterial burden and infection: the story of NERDS and STONES.* Advances in Skin & Wound Care, 19(8), 447–461. https://niche.org

Singh, A. (2023). Pitting Edema: What Is It, Causes, Grading, Diagnosis, Treatment, and More. https://www.osmosis.org/answers/pitting-edema

Sutton, J. (2020). *Erik Erikson's Stages of Psychosocial Development Explained.* https://positivepsychology.com/erikson-stages/

Yasir M, Mechanic OJ. (2023). *Syndrome of Inappropriate Antidiuretic Hormone Secretion.* : https://www.ncbi.nlm.nih.gov/books/NBK507777/

Wallace, D. (2006). *New Antinuclear Antibody Testing: Does it Cut Costs and Corners Without Jeopardizing Clinical Reliability?* https://www.medscape.com/viewarticle/543901_2

Weatherspoon, D. (2020). Metabolic Alkalosis. https://www.healthline.com/health/metabolic-alkalosis

World Health Organization. (2024). Sepsis. https://www.who.int/news-room/fact-sheets/detail/sepsis

World Health Organization. (2023). *Stroke, Cerebrovascular Accident.* https://www.emro.who.int/health-topics/stroke-cerebrovascular-accident/index.html.

www.ingramcontent.com/pod-product-compliance
Ingram Content Group UK Ltd.
Pitfield, Milton Keynes, MK11 3LW, UK
UKHW062013041026
15591UKWH00017B/1314